FATTY LIVER DIET

LIVE THE LIVER-FRIENDLY LIFESTYLE TO END OR AVOID NON-ALCOHOLIC FATTY LIVER DISEASE | YOUR COMPREHENSIVE GUIDE TO KNOW ALL ABOUT YOUR LIVER AND CREATE YOUR OWN LIVER-HEALTHY DIET

JUDY ROSE THOMPSON

© Copyright 2022 - All rights reserved.

The content contained within this book may not be reproduced, duplicated or transmitted without direct written permission from the author or the publisher.

Under no circumstances will any blame or legal responsibility be held against the publisher, or author, for any damages, reparation, or monetary loss due to the information contained within this book, either directly or indirectly.

Legal Notice:

This book is copyright protected. It is only for personal use. You cannot amend, distribute, sell, use, quote or paraphrase any part, or the content within this book, without the consent of the author or publisher.

Disclaimer Notice:

Please note the information contained within this document is for educational and entertainment purposes only. All effort has been executed to present accurate, up to date, reliable, complete information. No warranties of any kind are declared or implied. Readers acknowledge that the author is not engaged in the rendering of legal, financial, medical or professional advice. The content within this book has been derived from various sources. Please consult a licensed professional before attempting any techniques outlined in this book.

By reading this document, the reader agrees that under no circumstances is the author responsible for any losses, direct or indirect, that are incurred as a result of the use of the information contained within this document, including, but not limited to, errors, omissions, or inaccuracies.

Contents

Introduction 1
PART I: 3
A Closer Look at Nonalcoholic Fatty Liver Diseases 3
Chapter 1 5
All About Your Liver 5
    Main Functions of the Liver 9
Chapter 2 11
Nonalcoholic Fatty Liver Disease 11
    The Progression of NAFLD 12
    Nonalcoholic Steatohepatitis 17
    Symptoms of NAFLD and NASH 17
Chapter 3: 20
Diagnosing and Treating Fatty Liver Disease 20
    What if My Blood Tests are Abnormal? 22
    How is Fatty Liver Disease Treated or Cured? 24
PART II: 26
A Holistic Multidisciplinary Approach to Treating Fatty
Liver Disease 26
Chapter 4: 28
Taking a Holistic Approach 28
    A Holistic View: The Pillars of Health and NAFLD 29
    Treating NAFLD With Alternative Medicine 34
        Whole Medicine Practices 35
PART III 48
Creating a Liver-Healthy Lifestyle 48
Chapter 5 50
Liver-Friendly Lifestyle Changes 50
    How to Build New Habits 51
    Upgrading Your Mindset 54
    Weight Loss 57

- Exercise 59
- PART IV 65
- Healing Fatty Liver Through Diet 65
- Chapter 6 67
- Creating Your Fatty-Liver Diet Plan 67
  - Lifestyle and Diet Changes 68
  - Your Liver-Healthy Diet: Foods to Include 73
  - Your Liver-Healthy Diet: Foods to Avoid 81
  - The Fatty Liver Diet Program 85
- PART V 88
- Cleanses and Detox for Fatty Liver 88
- Chapter 7 90
- Natural Remedies for Fatty Liver Disease 90
  - Liver Cleanses 91
  - Herbal and Other Supplements 96
- Part VI 102
- Seven Rules to Follow for a Healthy Liver 102
- Chapter 8 104
- Seven Steps to Prevent and Reverse Fatty Liver Disease 104
  - Seven Steps to Reverse NAFLD 105
- Conclusion 113
- References 116

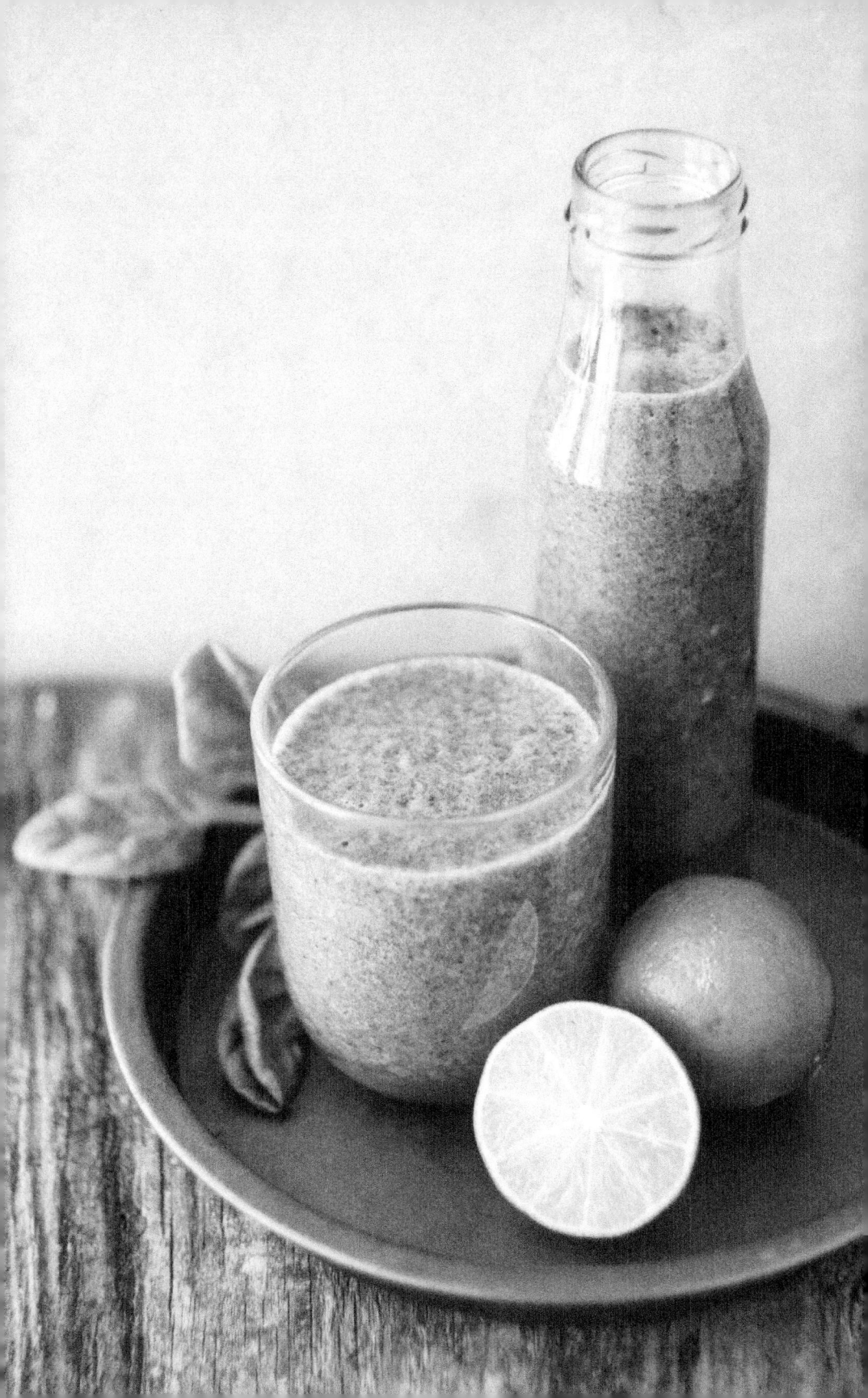

Introduction

The liver is known as the strong but silent organ. You know that it's there and that it's important to our survival, but you don't actually feel it working. It does its job behind the scenes, which is probably why the liver may be overlooked during the testing and diagnosis process when a person becomes ill. By the time more obvious symptoms of liver disease arise, the organ is already in distress and immediate medical intervention is required.

As strong as the liver is, it is also extremely vulnerable to damage, disease, and malfunction. One of its major functions is to filter harmful and toxic substances from the blood before they have the chance to be transmitted throughout the body via the bloodstream. The liver is like a bouncer for the body, making sure riffraff doesn't get past it and trash the place. It's important to remember that while a filter stops harmful substances from passing through, these toxins will leave a residue behind. The liver has a greater regenerative capacity than any other organ in the body. When that toxic residue lingers after it does its job, the liver can clean itself up so it's ready to tackle the next task. As resilient as the liver is, when its owner takes it for granted and abuses it, its superhero power of regeneration will slowly dissipate. If the liver's not able to function properly, the health of the whole body suffers. The conditions that result from liver damage range in severity from mild and reversible, to severe and incurable. There are forms of liver disease with a genetic cause, some are more environmentally-based (e.g. contracting hepatitis through exposure to the virus), and others are the result of lifestyle choices.

Whatever the determined cause, each diagnosis is unique, as is the way the disease is treated.

Receiving a diagnosis of liver disease, no matter the level of severity, comes with a complicated mix of emotions. It can be scary knowing that a vital organ you may never have given a second thought about before is in distress. It may cause self-blame–you may wonder how you could have let it get this far. But the situation isn't completely out of your control, and there are things you can do to get your health back on track.

The focus of this book is to prevent the worst-case scenario, and the best way to do that is to arm yourself with knowledge. The first step is to understand how the liver functions and what a healthy liver does for your body. The next step is to completely understand your condition, including the signs and symptoms specific to your form of liver disease and what you should or shouldn't be doing to improve and maintain your health. We'll also be looking at the treatments available for you, including natural and holistic options.

Nutrition and an overall healthy diet are crucial for the health of your liver. Yes, the liver does filter out the bad stuff, but it also helps to keep and distribute the good stuff too. Listening to the advice of a knowledgeable nutritionist and thinking about what you're putting into your body can make all the difference.

Living a healthy life with fatty liver disease doesn't have to be complicated. It comes down to three things: Stop consuming the things that directly harm your liver, switch to a healthy diet, and move your body every day.

That's the solid recipe for a healthy liver, and a healthier you

PART I:

A Closer Look at Nonalcoholic Fatty Liver Diseases

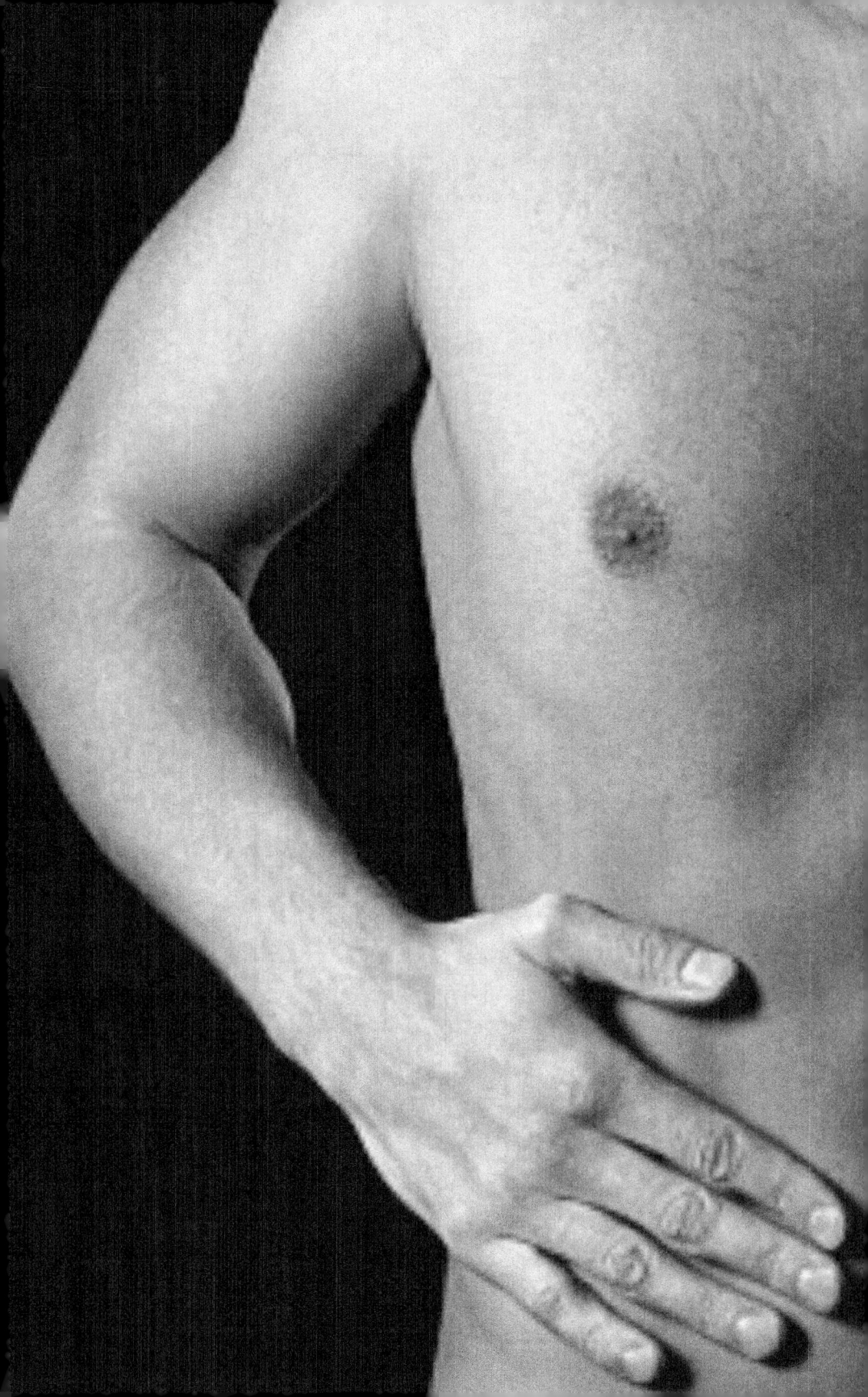

Chapter 1

All About Your Liver

Did you know that your liver performs over 500 functions in your body? As we said in the introduction, the liver is like a bouncer that stops harmful substances from traveling around the body in your bloodstream, but this is just one of its many functions. Understanding how a healthy liver works is essential to understanding the damage liver disease can do, and where the symptoms of liver disease come from. Arming yourself with knowledge also puts you at an advantage in your battle against liver disease. Since fatty liver disease is often invisible until the liver is damaged, being knowledgeable about the liver allows you to take action sooner, giving you a better chance of a full recovery. In this chapter, we'll focus on the general functions of the liver and how to maintain optimal liver health. This knowledge will be important to keep by your side when you start out on your journey to a healthier liver, and a healthier life overall. Anatomy of the Liver.

The liver is the largest solid internal organ as well as the largest gland in the body. This important organ is categorized as being part of the digestive system as it filters toxins from the blood, helps you to absorb and process nutrients from what you eat, and produces bile to eliminate harmful agents from the body. This is just the beginning of what your liver does for you!

The liver is located in the upper abdomen, just below the lungs at the bottom of the rib cage. This is what your physician gently pushes down on during a checkup to detect any swelling, tenderness, or the presence of any unusual masses. However, the only surefire way to confirm that the liver is in distress is to conduct blood work to check levels of liver enzymes in the blood–abnormal enzymes are a clear sign that something's wrong.

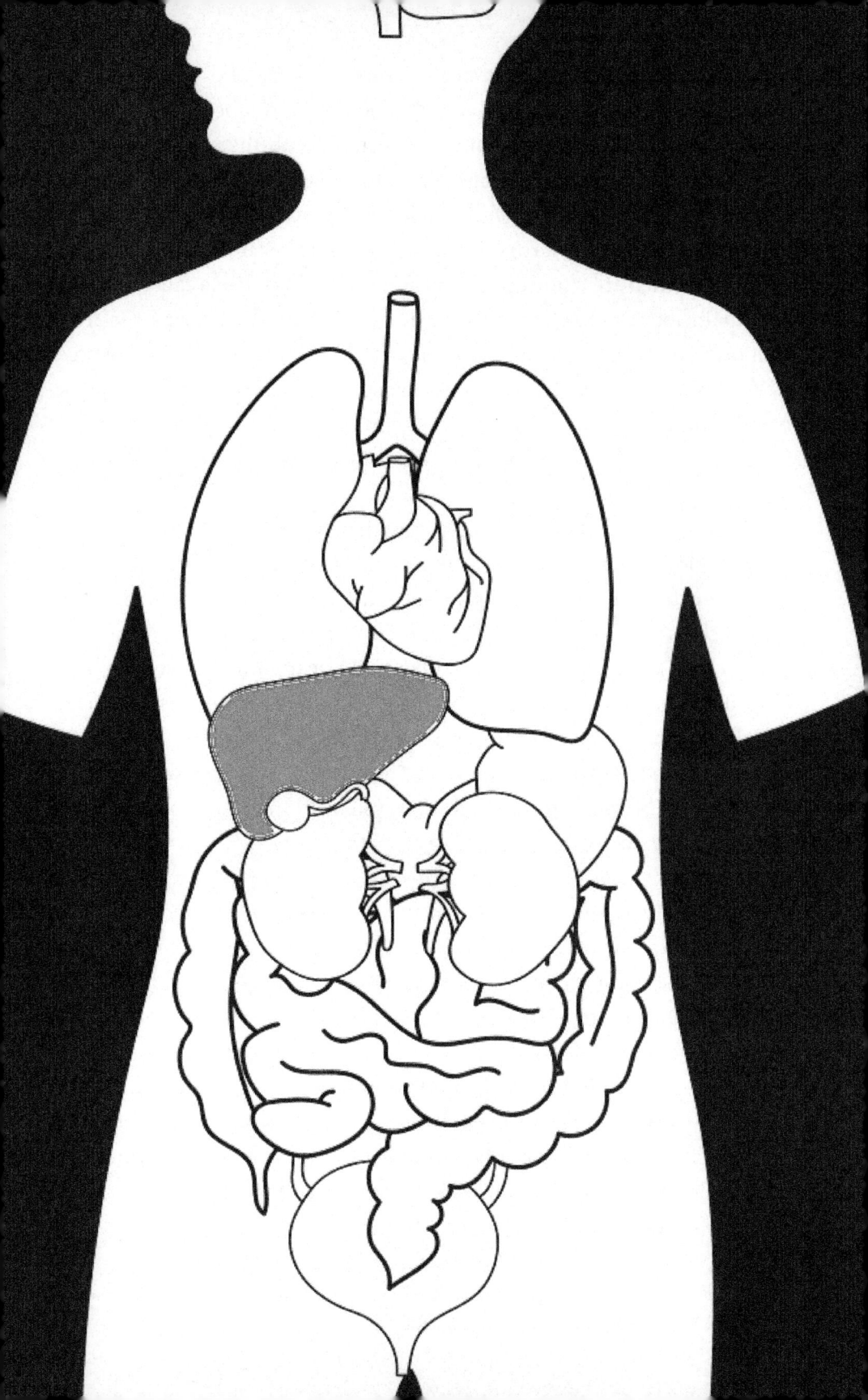

A healthy liver weighs in at around three to three-and-a-half pounds. It's roughly triangular in shape and divided into four lobes. The right and left lobes of the liver are the most important, with the smaller and less important caudate and quadrate lobes attached to the posterior or back side of the right lobe. These are called the accessory lobes, and aren't visible from the front. Across the four lobes, the liver is divided into eight segments, which are made up of thousands of small sections called lobules. The main lobes are separated by a band of tissue that keeps the liver anchored to the diaphragm, called the falciform ligament. This is covered by a fibrous tissue called Glisson's capsule, then further covered by a membrane called the visceral peritoneum. This double layer serves two purposes: holding the organ in place and protecting it from physical damage.

Because one of the liver's main functions is to filter toxins from the blood, blood flows into the organ through two vessels. The first is the hepatic portal vein which brings in nutrient-rich blood from the digestive system. This is the blood the liver filters for toxins. By contrast, the hepatic artery carries in oxygen-rich blood from the heart, which gives the liver cells the oxygen they need to do their jobs. Once the oxygen has been used up, deoxygenated blood exits through three hepatic veins, which are different from the hepatic portal vein. The hepatic veins also carry filtered, nutrient-rich blood from the digestive system to the heart to be stocked with oxygen before it is circulated around the body.

The main cells of the liver are called hepatocytes, and these are responsible for doing the actual filtering. These cells convert nutrients into compounds that are safe and accessible for the rest of your cells to absorb. If this didn't happen, the nutrients in your food would be either useless or harmful to your body's cells! Hepatocytes also take up toxins and make them safe for your body to get rid of without damaging itself. They may also metabolize compounds from your food into energy, so they can keep working. Finally, hepatocytes are responsible for synthesizing bile, which is needed for your body to digest fats. There are other kinds of cells in the liver, like Kuppfer cells, which guard the liver as part of the immune system.

Main Functions of the Liver

As we know, one of the foremost jobs the liver has is filtering unwanted compounds like toxins out of the blood. It also processes nutrients to make them safe and accessible for the rest of the body's cells. While the liver does a lot to remove harmful compounds from your blood, it adds useful compounds as well. One of these is albumin, which is the most common protein found in your blood. Albumin carries vitamins, minerals, and proteins around your body, while also preventing your blood from leaking out of blood vessels into the surrounding tissue. Remember albumin for later–it's part of the first blood test done to diagnose liver problems!

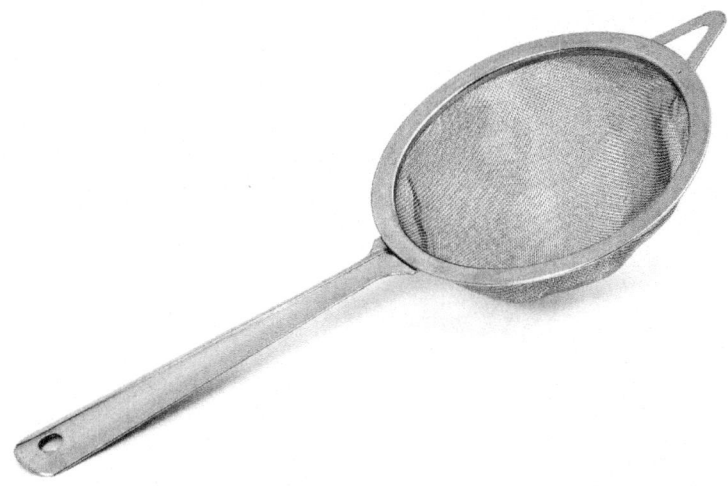

One of the other most important things your liver creates is a substance called bile, which is used to break down or emulsify fats in the intestines so you can absorb them. Bile also lets you absorb the fat-soluble vitamins A, D, E, and K, all of which are essential for your health. These vitamins, along with vitamin B12 and some minerals, are stored in the liver when there's extra in your food, allowing your body to keep functioning for some time if you have to go without.

Amino acids are commonly referred to as the building blocks of proteins, and amino acids from food are carried around the body in the blood. However, too much of some amino acids is toxic. The liver ensures that amino acids are at a healthy level in order to keep your cells and tissues safe. It also helps keep blood sugar at a healthy level, both by creating sugar via a process called gluconeogenesis and by removing excess sugar to store as glycogen. Glycogen is stored primarily in the liver and muscles, ready for your body to break it down whenever it needs energy in a pinch. Along with glucose, your liver can also synthesize fats, which can get out of control in some situations. Excess fat building up in the liver is at the core of nonalcoholic fatty liver disease (NAFLD). This will be more fully explained in the following chapters.

Now that you understand how the liver works, we can start talking about what happens when it doesn't work. In the next chapter, we'll look at NAFLD, the damage it does to your liver, and the tests doctors can use to diagnose it.

Chapter 2

Nonalcoholic Fatty Liver Disease

Liver disease isn't just one thing, but a big umbrella covering all the problems that could prevent the liver from performing its duties. This includes liver diseases caused by hepatitis viruses, liver disease caused by alcohol or drugs, genetic diseases, and more. Unlike many other forms of liver disease, NAFLD is unusual in that it has no known cause. While there are risk factors that can increase your odds of being diagnosed with NAFLD, there's no way to predict who will get it or not. One in four people live with some form of liver disease (Canadian Liver Foundation, n.d.). NAFLD is the most common liver disease, especially for those of us living in Western, fast-living, fast-eating parts of the world. Many of these cases are chronic, which means they continue over a long period of time. Unless your health is already in jeopardy, it usually takes a long time to develop liver disease. Generally, three quarters of the liver has to be affected before a decrease in its abilities becomes visible. Nonalcoholic liver disease and other liver disease can be slowed, stopped, or even reversed if they're caught early. But since the liver is so important, any kind of liver disease will have to be monitored for a lifetime once diagnosed. No matter how the disease is contracted, it's what you do from the point of diagnosis forward that makes a difference. In this chapter, we'll cover the progression of liver disease from inflammation (hepatitis) to liver cancer and the major symptoms you should never ignore.

The Progression of NAFLD

For many people, there are no obvious signs or symptoms of NAFLD at first, even if there is already damage to the liver. This is why it's important to bring up liver monitoring with your doctor at your regular checkup. In fact, simple liver enzyme tests aren't always included with routine blood work until there are signs there could be a concern. At that point, it might be too late to completely reverse the condition.

While there are over 100 forms of liver disease, most of them progress or worsen along the same pathway. If you've been diagnosed with NAFLD, it's important to familiarize yourself with these steps so that you can fully understand your doctor and what they're telling you.

There are a few things you need to understand about how liver disease develops before we can explore it further. At the center of these diseases is inflammation, a common type of immune reaction. Inflammation involves increasing blood flow, cranking up the heat, and sending cells and proteins from the immune system to the site of the infection or damage. This creates a hostile environment for invaders like bacteria, but if it becomes chronic, it can start to damage healthy cells and tissues instead. Inflammation in the liver is called hepatitis. Additionally, since the liver's main job is filtering out things the body doesn't need or that could be potentially harmful, sometimes residue is left behind.

An example is when you go out and overdo it with rich foods and alcohol and then wake up feeling really lousy. This comes from the liver telling you to take it easy, because it's working hard to undo the damage from the night before. If you don't give the organ the recovery time it needs and keep putting it through the same thing, it's going to start wearing out. There's only so much it can take! The residue building up in the liver from abuse, as well as fat buildup in the liver, can both contribute to inflammation. Steatosis is the medical name for inflammation caused by fat buildup in the liver, and nonalcoholic steatosis is the medical name for when this occurs in people with NAFLD. We'll talk more about nonalcoholic steatosis later.

Compared to hepatitis, fibrosis is a more dangerous stage of liver disease, which comes from an excess of collagen, a common structural protein in human bodies. When your liver is inflamed, your cells produce a lot of collagen in order to repair damage. This works great when there's an actual infection causing the inflammation, but if the inflammation is chronic, the collagen builds up and the liver begins to scar. Scar tissue in the liver can get in the way of blood flow, starving liver cells of the oxygen they need to do their jobs. The liver can't regenerate cells to replace useless scar tissue, so if fibrosis continues, the liver won't be able to function. Fibrosis can be reversed in earlier stages, but if left too long it can result in cirrhosis, which is much more serious.

When the liver becomes severely scarred and permanently damaged, doctors call this stage cirrhosis. As mentioned above, the liver can't regenerate or replace scar tissue, which means that cirrhosis is irreversible. However, it can be slowed if caught early enough. Cirrhosis can also lead to a number of other dangerous complications, such as portal hypertension, which is when scarring blocks blood from draining into the liver from the digestive system and the liver can't filter out harmful compounds. This can lead to hepatic encephalopathy, which is when ammonia in the bloodstream is not filtered out and starts to interfere with brain function. Another serious complication is ascites, which is when fluid from the liver seeps out into the abdomen. This causes a lot of pain and discomfort, and sometimes the swelling is even visible from outside the body.

Finally, advanced liver disease can increase your odds of developing cancer. If you've been diagnosed with liver disease, your physician or natural health provider should help you arrange regular ultrasounds to monitor the progression of cirrhosis as well as to check for any signs of cancer. Staying on top of any changes in overall health, as well as monitoring for symptoms of liver disease, should be a regular step in maintaining well-being. If you aren't doing what's best for your liver, it can't do what's best for you.

Why is NAFLD Becoming More Common?

Scientists haven't figured out where NAFLD really comes from–it doesn't have a clear cause the way that alcohol-related fatty liver disease does. Genetics, obesity, and an inflammatory diet have all been suggested as possible causes of the disease, but it's impossible to predict who will get the disease and who won't. In this section, we'll talk about the major risk factors for NAFLD, and which people are more likely than others to develop it. Being obese or overweight is a very common risk factor for NAFLD, and the fact that more and more people are becoming obese or overweight every year is one of the main reasons that more and more people are being diagnosed with NAFLD. Diseases that are more common in people who are obese, such as type II diabetes, high blood pressure, and high cholesterol are also linked to NAFLD. In 1999-2000, 30.5% of Americans were suffering from obesity, while in 2017-2018, that percentage had risen to 42.4% (Centers for Disease Control and Prevention, n.d.-b).

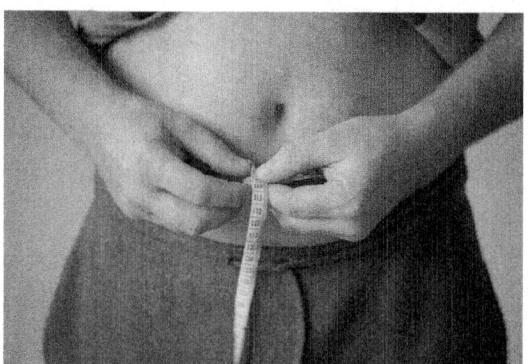

Obesity contributes to NAFLD by increasing the amount of fat your liver produces. Your liver breaks down fats for energy, and also produces them to send to the rest of your body. There are many reasons that your liver would be synthesizing fats and fatty acids. For example, if you have extra sugar in the blood, your liver will take those up to store as glycogen. However, your body can only store so much glycogen at a time, and if stores are full, your body knows it's time to start synthesizing triglycerides, or fat, instead. This is how weight gain occurs if that stored fat isn't burnt off. While this is part of the reason that NAFLD is becoming more common, it's not the end of the story, and plenty of people within a healthy weight range are also diagnosed with the disease.

The prevalence of fast-food and packaged snacks is another potential reason that NAFLD is becoming more common. For many of us, it's easy to get our hands on unhealthy foods–between fast-food, vending machines, and delivery, many people can be snacking minutes after they think of it! These snacks are often high in saturated trans fats, refined sugars, and sodium, which can contribute to a number of health problems and may be linked to NAFLD; these foods are often addictive and high in calories, which makes it easier to put on extra weight. There's one more reason that junk food is linked to NAFLD, and that's fructose. Fructose is a type of sugar found in fruits and fruit juices, as well as anything that has high-fructose corn syrup, a common sweetener in sodas, fruity drinks, and packaged treats. Your liver uses fructose to synthesize fats and fatty acids that your body needs, and this is a normal, vital function! The only issue is that fructose isn't just an ingredient: it actually starts this process. When there is too much fructose in the diet, the liver will just continue making fatty substances that have nowhere to go, until they build up. A diet high in fructose is linked to NAFLD even if you're not obese, so once again don't assume you're safe just because your weight is under control!

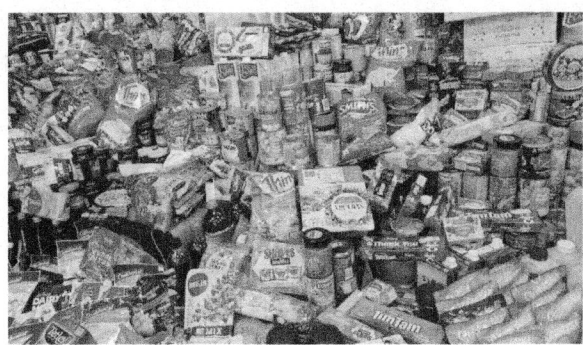

Finally, our lifestyles are becoming less and less active, especially as indoor, sit-down entertainment like video games become more popular. Not only that, but with the rise of automation, our jobs and careers involve less and less physical activity as time goes on. Something else making us more sedentary than before is the cost of living. As necessities and luxuries become more expensive, it gets more difficult to take up sports or other types of physical activity that cost money. For the same reason, people are also moving out of the city and living in nearby suburbs, meaning they spend more time sitting in their car during their commute each day. While being very sedentary contributes to obesity, it's also a risk factor for NAFLD on its own, and one possible reason that people who don't suffer from obesity still develop the disease.

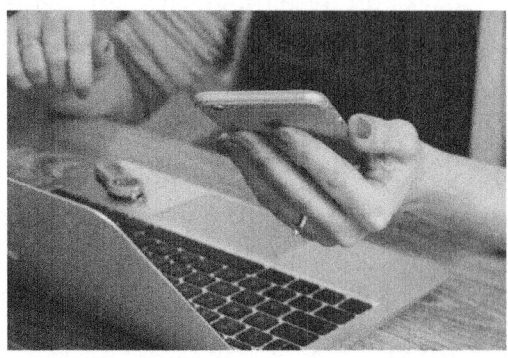

Some populations are more likely to be diagnosed with NAFLD than others. This is commonly thought to be due to genetics. For example, people who are Hispanic are more likely than other groups to have NAFLD while African-Americans are much less likely to be diagnosed. Genetics may also play a role in people who carry fat primarily around the abdomen and people with polycystic ovary syndrome being more at risk for NAFLD. Other risk factors include being exposed to toxins, taking certain medications like corticosteroids, being malnourished, and having hormonal issues like hypothyroidism. Finally, age is another risk factor. While kids can get NAFLD in rare cases, the disease is much more common in people who are middle-aged or older, possibly because they've been making certain lifestyle choices for a longer time.

NAFLD refers simply to the buildup of fats in the liver, but when left unchecked this can lead to nonalcoholic steatohepatitis (NASH), which we'll discuss next. Being aware of the lifestyle choices that can contribute to NAFLD, as well as any possible risk factors you might carry, gives you the best possible chance to catch and treat NAFLD before it progresses to NASH.

Nonalcoholic Steatohepatitis

If you are diagnosed with NASH, it means that the fatty deposits in the liver have become inflamed and scarring has started. The word "steatohepatitis" is a combination of "steatosis" (fatty buildup in the liver) and "hepatitis" (chronic inflammation of the liver). NASH is much more serious than NAFLD; it can become life-threatening without careful medical attention. Despite this, early-stage cases may not have symptoms, and many people don't realize they have it. On top of this, not everyone with NAFLD will eventually develop NASH, making it even harder to predict when this frightening condition will strike.

It's suggested that 1.5-6.45% of the world's population lives with NASH (The NASH Education Program, n.d.) but it's likely that this number is lower than the reality. Diagnosing NASH is even more difficult than diagnosing NAFLD, as doctors need to do a liver biopsy to confirm the diagnosis. This is a much more invasive procedure than a simple blood test, as the physician must remove a small piece of the liver for examination and testing. In most cases, neither of these are done until symptoms appear, meaning that most detected cases are more advanced.

The early symptoms (pain and discomfort in the abdomen and persistent fatigue) are commonly found in milder gastrointestinal illnesses, making it even harder to catch NASH early on. The next section covers the common symptoms of NAFLD and NASH, which we hope will make it easier for our readers to spot their symptoms and ask their doctors to check on their liver health.

Symptoms of NAFLD and NASH

Recall that while there's over 100 known forms of liver disease, they often progress in very similar ways. In this vein, there's also a list of common symptoms that apply to a vast range of liver diseases, as well as other conditions not related to the liver! However, having several of the symptoms discussed below is definitely a reason to ask your doctor for blood work to check up on your liver; it's much better to be safe than sorry! There are a lot of symptoms that are milder and could easily go ignored if you don't know what to look for. Make no mistake: Even though these symptoms don't seem very serious, any symptoms of a liver problem are a clear sign the liver is in active distress. These include skin itchiness, rashes or redness, swelling around the feet, legs, and ankles, unusual bruising, unexplained weight loss, fever or chills, sore joints and muscles, fatigue, dry eyes and mouth, and unexplained nausea.

Other symptoms are more serious and could indicate that you're dealing with liver problems or another severe condition. For example, if you feel a mass in your abdomen, that's something that should never be ignored. This could be a sign that your liver is swelling from inflammation. A sudden personality change, such as becoming much more aggressive or having unexplained memory issues, could be a sign that toxins in your blood are affecting your brain.

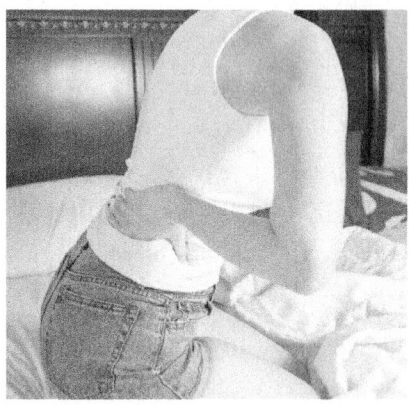

There are a few symptoms of NAFLD and NASH that more clearly indicate that there's something wrong with your liver. Jaundice, which is when the skin and the whites of the eyes take on a distinct yellowish color, is a major symptom of advanced NAFLD and advanced NASH. This happens when your liver isn't filtering your blood properly, causing a toxic substance called bilirubin to build up. Another sign of high bilirubin is dark urine when you're not dehydrated. If you're drinking plenty of water and your urine is still taking on a deep yellow or brown color, it's time to seek medical attention. Finally, abdominal swelling when you're not pregnant or bloated can be a sign that fluid from the liver is building up in the abdomen. This needs to be seen and treated by a doctor as soon as possible.

Our next chapter will cover how fatty liver disease is diagnosed, the kinds of professionals to have on your liver team, and your options for treatment. The most important thing to remember is that you shouldn't be alone in your battle against this disease–your medical team is there to guide you through this frightening time and help you find the treatments that are best for you.

Chapter 3:

Diagnosing and Treating Fatty Liver Disease

The process of getting diagnosed with a liver condition can be a difficult one. Remember that when you first arrive at the doctor with unexplained symptoms, you might not get a diagnosis right away. The doctor needs to rule out the most common conditions first. It can be extremely frustrating to go through this process, but sticking with it is essential to getting the right diagnosis.

While they do need to rule out more common conditions, your doctor also has a responsibility to fully investigate the symptoms you're experiencing. They should listen closely to your concerns, and if you're experiencing symptoms of NAFLD, order a blood test panel. If your doctor doesn't listen to your concerns and conduct a thorough investigation, get a second opinion. The health of your liver is extremely important, so don't be afraid to advocate for yourself and your needs! In this section, we'll be covering the various tests that are usually conducted in determining the kind of liver disease you may be living with, and the lifestyle changes that are usually recommended as treatment.Blood Enzyme Tests

While there may be a physical examination and some additional tests first, one of the most important parts of diagnosing a liver condition is the blood enzyme tests. The levels of different enzymes, or proteins, in the blood will not only help tell if the liver is in distress, but can also hint at how serious the situation is. Some damage may not be visible on an ultrasound, but if blood work reveals that your liver is failing to filter waste from the blood, it's clear that something's wrong.

The first test is the albumin test. As we know, albumin is synthesized in and secreted from your liver on a daily basis. Low albumin is a bad sign as a healthy liver naturally keeps this in normal range. Alanine transaminase (ALT), another important enzyme in the liver, is also tested. ALT leaks out of damaged liver cells, and people with NAFLD may have high levels in their blood. You'll also get the ALP test, which examines how much alkaline phosphatase is present in your blood. When levels of ALP are abnormal, it's usually a sign there is something wrong with the liver, gallbladder, or kidneys.

There are several other enzymes not specific to your liver that are included in blood enzyme tests. Abnormal levels of these enzymes combined with the tests above can help your doctor determine a diagnosis. These include aspartate transaminase (AST), gamma-glutamyl transferase (GGT), and L-lactate dehydrogenase (LDH).

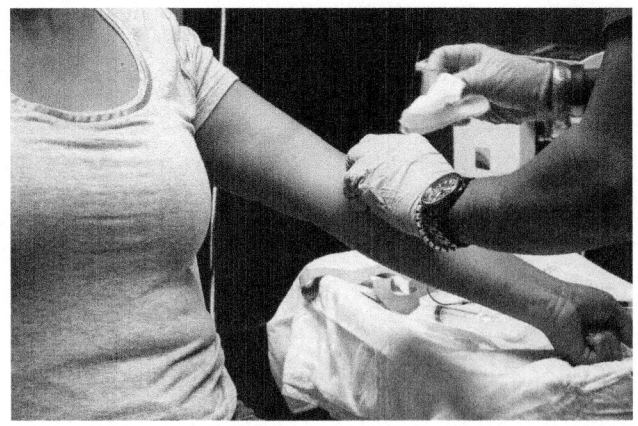

Finally, not every blood test checks levels of an enzyme. Bilirubin, which we've mentioned before, is a yellow-tinged waste product produced when old red blood cells break down. When bilirubin levels are high, it could indicate that your liver isn't properly filtering the blood.

What if My Blood Tests are Abnormal?

If the levels of liver enzymes in your blood are abnormal, your medical team will investigate further to see if your liver is in trouble or if there's another explanation. For example, there are certain prescribed medications or viral infections that could alter blood levels of liver enzymes. If there's no other explanation, your doctor may decide more serious testing is needed. While these tests can seem scary, in most cases you will only have to undergo a couple of them to determine whether you have liver disease, and how advanced it is.

An abdominal ultrasound is a simple procedure where the technologist uses a wand-like instrument on the outside of your abdomen to take pictures of your liver and other organs from different angles. This is usually first on the list of tests after the blood enzyme tests. The technologist may also take a recording of blood flow to and from the liver to see if there's a blockage, or test for stiffness (elastography) to see if fibrosis has started. Elastography is done by measuring sound waves as they pass through the liver tissue.

The abdominal computed tomography (CT) scan is an upgraded version of the regular ultrasound. Usually the patient takes a contrast dye into their body to highlight the organs for a clearer image. Most often, this dye is administered by injection in order to view solid organs such as the liver, but if other organs are included, the dye may also be given orally or through an enema, depending on your individual case. A CT scan allows the doctor to see cross-sections of the liver, in case the damage is only visible inside the organ. A CT machine is donut-shaped, and the embedded camera spins around the patient's body to take pictures. CT scans are usually painless, though if you're having dye injected you may feel a pinch from the needle. The dye can also make you feel warm or put a weird taste in your mouth, but don't worry: this will pass after the procedure.

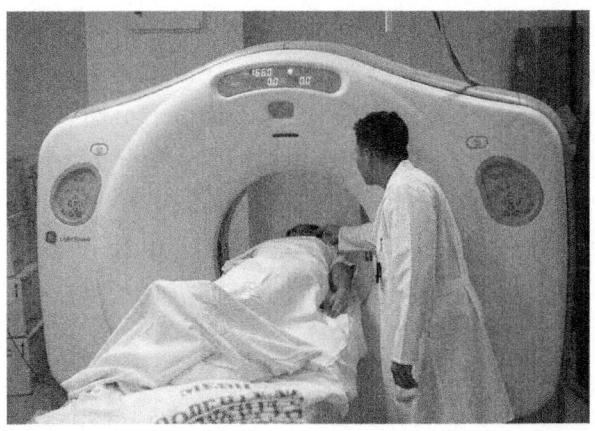

A magnetic resonance imagery (MRI) scan is a more advanced type of CT scan that creates more detailed images for the specialist to analyze. MRI scans don't hurt and there's no dye injection, but some patients find the 45-60 minute procedure scary if they are afraid of enclosed spaces or loud noises. If you're nervous, remember that you'll be able to speak to the technologist through a PA system the entire time, so they'll know if you're in distress.

So what happens if an ultrasound, CT scan, or MRI scan shows there's a problem? In that case, your doctor might order a liver biopsy. This is a slightly more invasive procedure where, using a long needle, a tiny piece of the liver is removed and examined with a microscope. A liver biopsy is usually needed to confirm a diagnosis of NASH. Local anesthetic is given during the biopsy to make you more comfortable, and your doctor may prescribe some pain medication for afterwards as well.

How is Fatty Liver Disease Treated or Cured?

Once testing is complete, your doctor will be able to start putting together a treatment plan specific to your needs. If NAFLD is detected early and if you make the necessary lifestyle changes as soon as possible, the condition has a high chance of being reversed. In more severe cases where the patient has been diagnosed with NASH, the focus will be on stopping or slowing the progress of the damage. There are currently no approved medications that can help with NAFLD, but that doesn't mean you're helpless. Making lifestyle changes, such as taking up a special diet and an exercise regimen, are the first weapons in your arsenal when it comes to fighting NAFLD and NASH. Some alternative medical practices include treatments that proponents believe can help fight NAFLD, and an open-minded traditional doctor, holistic doctor, or naturopath can help connect you to these options. You may also want to look into cleanses or herbal supplements. Finally, your doctor might prescribe medication to help you manage your symptoms, or to make up for a loss of liver function.

In the absolute most severe cases of cirrhosis, a liver transplant may be called for, but this is rare! If your disease has progressed to this point, your doctor can inform you on how the process of getting matched with a donor works in your area, and what steps to take in the meantime. Most NAFLD and NASH cases don't require a transplant, and instead a lifestyle-based treatment is much more common. However, the specific goals can change depending on the person.

Losing weight, usually three to five percent of total body weight, is the most common recommendation for people with NAFLD. If you're underweight or happen to be suffering from poor nutrition, your doctor or other medical professionals can advise you as to how to fix this without adding more unwanted fat to your liver. Regardless of your weight, you'll also likely be asked to cut out harmful foods containing a lot of sodium, refined carbs, fructose, and saturated fats, as all of these components can harm your liver. Even if the goal isn't to lose weight, exercise is a common component of most NAFLD treatment plans as it helps metabolize fats.

Depending on your individual case, your doctor might have other instructions you may not have realized are relevant to your liver health. This can include managing chronic illnesses like diabetes and high blood pressure that can increase inflammation and thus worsen NAFLD. You may also be asked to reduce your stress levels and get better sleep, as both of these steps are essential for managing inflammation and improving your general health. Your doctor will most likely also ask you to avoid alcohol at all costs. While alcohol isn't the cause of NAFLD, it's very harmful to a damaged liver, and will only make things worse!

So if you take all of these steps seriously, how long does it take to recover from NAFLD? Unfortunately, the answer once again depends on your individual situation. Your doctor may assign you a grade that indicates how advanced your condition is. If you follow lifestyle changes to the letter, grade 1 can be reversed in a couple of months. Grade 2 is more concerning, but can be reversed in 10-20 months if you're diligent. Unfortunately, grade 3 is assigned to people with more serious scarring and damage, when the disease is too advanced to be completely reversed. Some people with grade 3 liver disease can gradually recover over several years, but stopping or slowing the progress of damage is all that can be done in most of these cases.

Remember that the liver will be as kind to you as you are to it: This resilient organ usually responds well to a healthy lifestyle, and will begin to regenerate if the damage isn't too advanced. If you take the reins of your treatment and take initiative to live a healthier life, you're doing exactly what you need to do to manage your NAFLD.

PART II:

A Holistic Multidisciplinary Approach to Treating Fatty Liver Disease

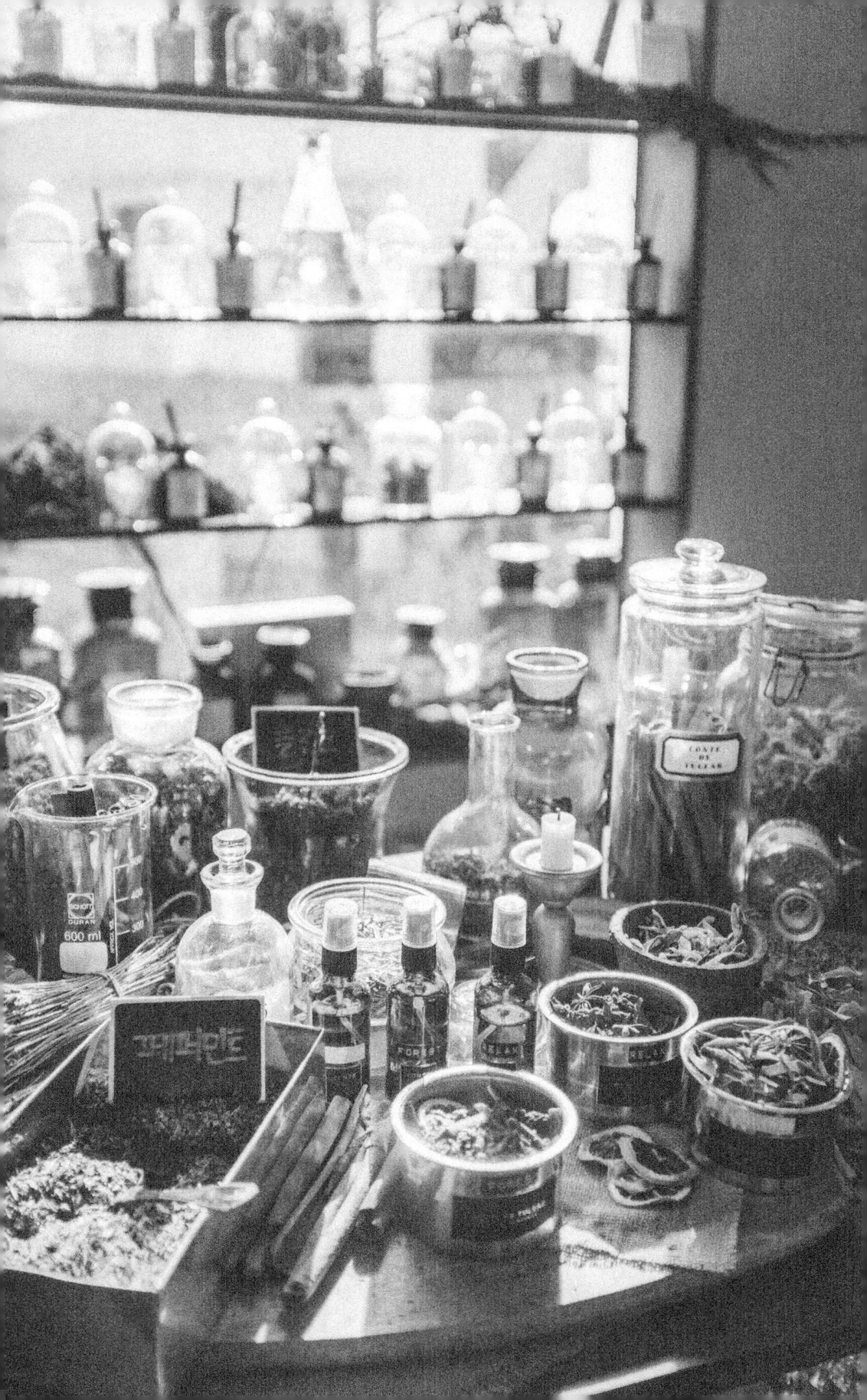

Chapter 4:

Taking a Holistic Approach

What is holistic medicine, and how does it differ from traditional medicine? Traditional medicine tends to focus on one organ system or one problem at a time. On the other hand, holistic medicine teaches that you can't just treat one part of a patient: Since all organ systems are connected, the patient needs to be treated as a whole person. When one area isn't being tended to the way it should be, the whole suffers.

Holistic doctors are your best bet when it comes to accessing this kind of treatment plan. When an individual seeks the help of a holistic physician, they tap into both traditional and alternative forms of healthcare to give the patient the best treatment possible. In the case of a person with NAFLD, for example, the holistic practitioner would not ignore the results of blood enzyme tests and ultrasounds, as well as any medication the patient was prescribed, while also investigating natural options for treatment as well as lifestyle changes. In some cases, they may suggest a regimen of herbal supplements, or a visit to a reiki practitioner or acupuncturist to accompany the lifestyle changes recommended by the primary physician.

In this section, we'll cover generally what holistic medicine is, the ways the holistic approach can help, what it can't promise to help, and how to incorporate holistic medicine into your liver health plan. We'll also touch on the basics of some popular alternative medicine practices and what they can do for your liver health if you've been diagnosed with NAFLD.

A Holistic View: The Pillars of Health and NAFLD

Every person with NAFLD is unique, and so every treatment plan is unique. A treatment plan for a person who needs to lose weight, for example, would be different from that of a person whose concern is malnutrition or who is at the advanced NASH or cirrhosis stage.

Up to this point, the goal has been to guide you through the medical jargon so you can understand both NAFLD and NASH without having to spend years in medical school. If you can communicate your needs to your medical team, you're much better equipped to help them help you. The wonderful thing about the holistic view of medicine is that rather than sticking to just one path to turn your health around, you're able to take bits and pieces from a variety of sources that work together with your needs.

Before moving forward, it's important to know the difference among traditional, holistic, and naturopathic medicines. A traditional practitioner is the image of the doctor working in clinics and hospitals. They don't eliminate alternative options, but focus on Western medicine and prescription medications. The naturopathic practitioner has done the same rigorous medical degree program as the traditional doctor and is capable of prescribing medication; however, their main perspective is on self-healing and examining natural methods of healing. Finally, the holistic practitioner combines methods from both modern and natural medical fields together to bring their patients the benefits of each.

The holistic physician or alternative medicine practitioner taps into different areas that affect human health to help create a balance among them. These are called the pillars of health. While traditional or Western medicine focuses mainly on physical and sometimes mental health, the holistic view goes much further. Learning the pillars of health can help you determine where the problem is so you can fix it. Depending on your unique situation and the holistic provider's school of thought (there are many forms of alternative medicine!), there can be different numbers of pillars they will address. The main five are physical health, mental health, emotional health, social health, and spiritual health, and some practitioners add in nutritional, financial, and occupational health as well.

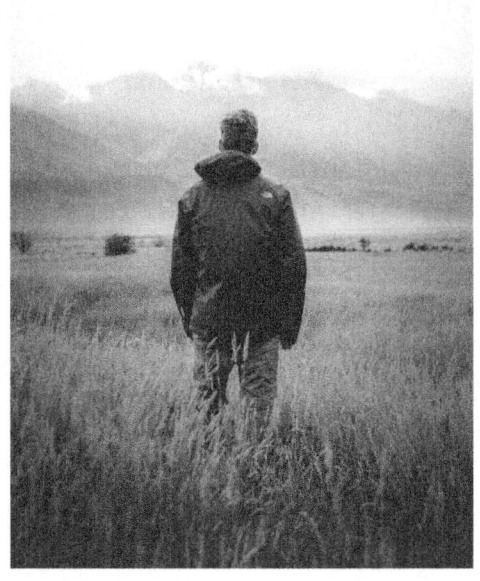

When discussing our health, the physical body is the first thing that comes to mind. We usually notice what affects our physical health before anything else. This includes getting enough sleep, getting enough exercise, and limiting how many toxins we take in through drinking, smoking, and other harmful habits. It can also include eating a varied and healthy diet, though sometimes this is covered under the nutritional pillar of health instead. Falling short in any of these areas not only puts your health in general at risk, but also increases your risk for NAFLD directly or indirectly. For example, not getting enough exercise and eating a poor diet can increase your risk of NAFLD if you become overweight. Eating a diet high in saturated fats and fructose can also encourage fat to build up in your liver. Not getting enough sleep can affect your liver in a more indirect manner, as getting less sleep increases your risk of being overweight and of suffering from type II diabetes or heart disease, both of which are linked to NAFLD as well (Mir et al., 2013).

The next pillar of health from the holistic viewpoint is mental health. Although mental health is often grouped with emotional health, in holistic medicine they're treated separately. Emotional health concerns how your mood and emotions are impacted throughout your day, while mental health focuses more on your thoughts, understanding, and cognitive functioning. For people used to thinking about health in a traditional way, it may be unclear how mental health and the liver are associated. The liver can affect the brain–when a liver is not filtering toxins from the blood, the toxins can build up and begin to affect the brain, causing confusion and other neurological symptoms. The relationship can go the other way as well. Mental illnesses such as depression and anxiety are linked to increased inflammation throughout the body, and while more research needs to be done to confirm the link, it's very possible that poor mental health can put you at risk for NAFLD or vice versa (Shea et al., 2021).

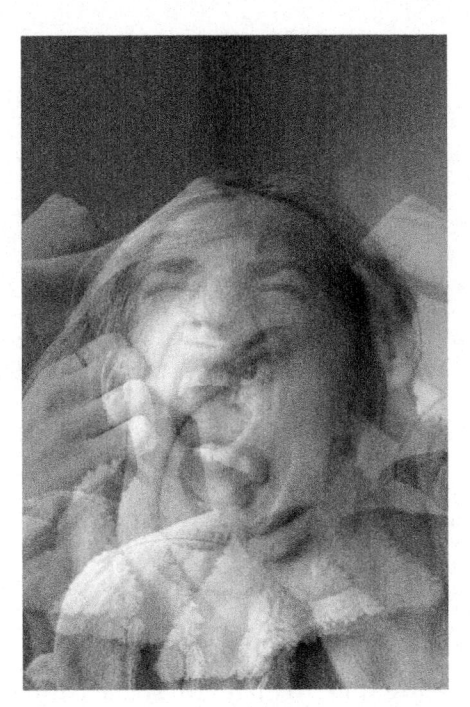

Emotional health is closely connected to both physical and mental health, and can also affect your liver. Since our emotions cause different physical reactions, such as an elevated heart rate or higher levels of different hormones, the emotions we feel can affect our physical body. The biggest concern here is stress, which can increase inflammation and put you at risk for health problems like type II diabetes that are linked to NAFLD. So how do we manage stress? The key is not to develop the ability to control what you're feeling, but more to control how you respond to people and situations. We face stressors every day. It's important to be in tune with what you're feeling and how you respond to situations so you can learn to cope with those stressors more effectively. Remember that chronic stress can exacerbate inflammation, including in the liver. Furthermore, in some alternative medicine practices such as traditional Chinese medicine, the liver is deeply connected to emotion, and taking care of your emotional well-being will be an intrinsic part of your liver health plan.

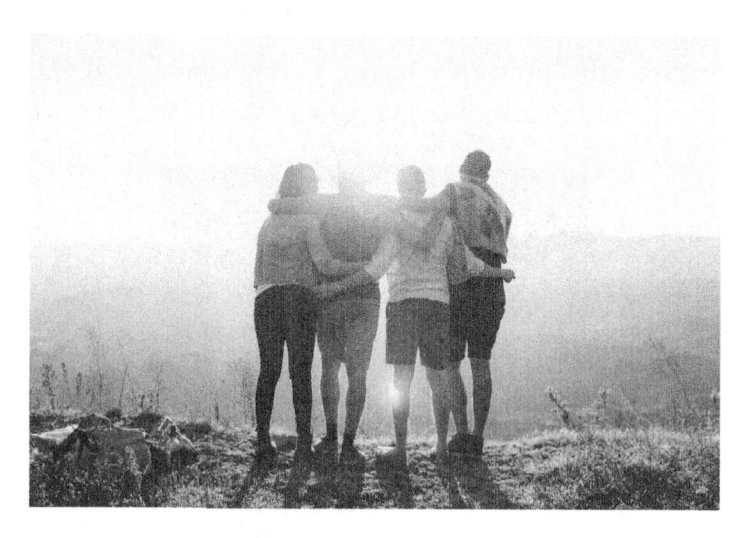

You may not realize the importance of your social life to your health, but it's much easier to get through tough days when you have a connection with family, friends and other people who support you. Being isolated can increase anxiety, stress, or other conditions that may be linked to NAFLD. During the COVID-19 pandemic, social connection became extremely difficult. But regardless of your situation and whether you're coping with quarantine, there are still ways to maintain social connection while staying safe. In these modern times, social media, cell phones, and other ways to video chat can help. Reaching out to volunteer in the community, even remotely, is socially comforting. While it's important to keep those positive people close, be sure to keep a distance from those who cause you anxiety or unnecessary stress. When dealing with NAFLD, you don't need additional toxicity in your life, and it's much easier to make the lifestyle changes needed to improve your health when you're surrounded by supportive people.

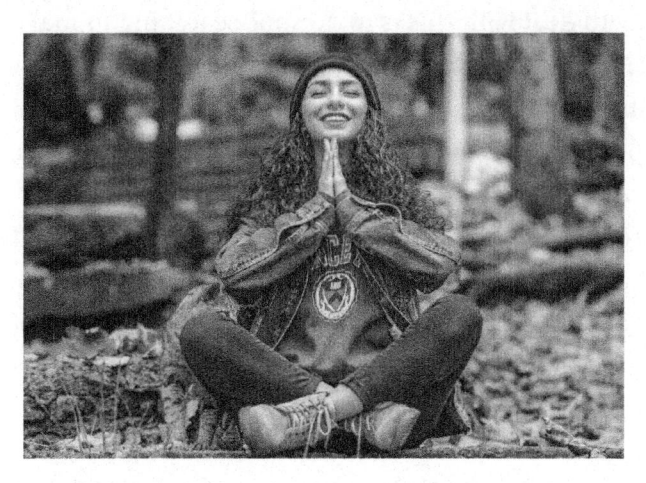

Finally, spiritual well-being is also worth looking into. Some people see being spiritual as being religious. While religion can be part of a spiritual practice, it's not the only thing that matters. The key is connecting to the core of yourself and believing in something outside of yourself. If you have trouble connecting with your spiritual side, try spending time in nature. Take a walk in the woods, sit by a waterfall, or float in water. If you are religious, give yourself time each day to practice your beliefs. Prayer, meditation, and worship can all be helpful here. Your spiritual health is important when struggling with NAFLD because spirituality elicits hope and helps build your inner strength to fight for your liver and your overall health. Being spiritually connected can also help reduce anxiety and stress.

There are three more pillars of health that your holistic practitioner might address. The first is nutritional, which we touched on within the physical pillar and will be covered in more detail in the rest of the book. Another is the financial pillar. When finances are a major concern, you'll definitely be coping with stress and worry that affects your well-being. Seeking the help of a financial advisor can help you get this area back under your control. There are specific resources for patient groups that can assist you physically and financially. For example, there are volunteer ride-share offerings for appointments, state-run home-care services, and discounted prescription-based exercise programs that can reduce the financial burden of accessing appropriate healthcare. The eighth pillar is occupational. Your job can be the source of a lot of joy, or a lot of stress. The best way to deal with this is to do soul-searching to make sure you're doing something you find fulfilling, and explore ways to get work done in a less stressful environment.

The key is to reduce as much outside stress, negativity, and worry as you have control over so that you can concentrate on what's most important right now: the health of your liver. If you feel ready, read over this outline of the holistic pillars and write down what you want to go into more detail about with your primary healthcare provider. They may have suggestions for where to get started, or be able to connect you with resources to help you on your way.

Treating NAFLD With Alternative Medicine

Traditional or Western medicine doesn't have all the answers, so many people look to alternative therapies as part of their treatment plan for a range of different reasons. Obviously, many people are looking to alternative methods to cure their health problems, including NAFLD, where they feel like traditional medicine can't. While alternative medical practices can be helpful additions to your treatment plan, it's important not to focus on them to the exclusion of traditional medicine. Your best chance to improve your condition lies in listening to the advice of your primary physician, and working with them to incorporate alternative practices into your treatment. Remember, a good doctor will be open-minded and willing to work with you to get you the treatment you need!

That point made, there are additional reasons that liver patients look into alternative medicine. These treatments can boost energy and motivation by fostering a positive outlook. Feeling like you're able to do something about your condition can help motivate you to keep fighting, and having a choice in your treatment options is very empowering. Alternative options may also work to reduce the severity of your symptoms through their physical effects on your body, such as reducing inflammation. If you're concerned about toxins in medication, finding natural or alternative ways to manage your symptoms can be very comforting. Finally, alternative medicine can strengthen the immune system. This is a huge bonus for liver patients whose immune systems are highly compromised.

Last of all, please don't view traditional and alternative medicine as enemies, or feel like you can only pick one or the other! Many traditional doctors encourage their patients to explore alternative medicine. There are many different types of complementary and alternative practices to choose from, so it's important to research each to find what you'd feel most comfortable incorporating into your treatment plan. If you aren't getting what you expect from one, or if it makes you feel uncomfortable or worsens any of your symptoms, there's no shame in trying something else. Remember that every case is unique! Tap into the insight of your primary health care provider to see which practices they feel match your personal goals. Next, we'll discuss different kinds of alternative medicine and what they can do for your liver health. This can be a great jumping-off point to determine which kind of alternative medicine is right for you.

Whole Medicine Practices

These practices blend herbal and other natural forms of medicine with cultural beliefs that have been practiced for centuries or even millenia. Being forms of holistic medicine, whole medicine practices treat the body as a whole, instead of as a group of parts. Three of the most widely recognized forms of whole medicine are naturopathy, traditional Chinese medicine (TCM), and Ayurvedic medicine.

Naturopathy

Naturopathy is a well-rounded school of thought on how to treat health problems that mixes modern and alternative methods. The key is using as many natural and non-toxic materials as possible to promote healing. Naturopathic doctors have legitimate medical degrees and are able to provide medication to people who need them, but their involvement goes much further than that. They also focus on working out which lifestyle changes need to be made in order to get the patient's health back on track, how the patient might be able to reduce their stress, and may also recommend a regimen of herbs and dietary supplements to support the patient's health. Naturopathic doctors can also administer or direct the patient towards other alternative medical treatments including homeopathy, and manipulative therapies such as chiropractic. They may recommend counseling or another form of mental health care if a patient's mental health is suffering. Finally, naturopaths will sometimes guide the patient through a cleanse or detox, making them excellent additions to your team if a liver cleanse is something you're interested in doing.

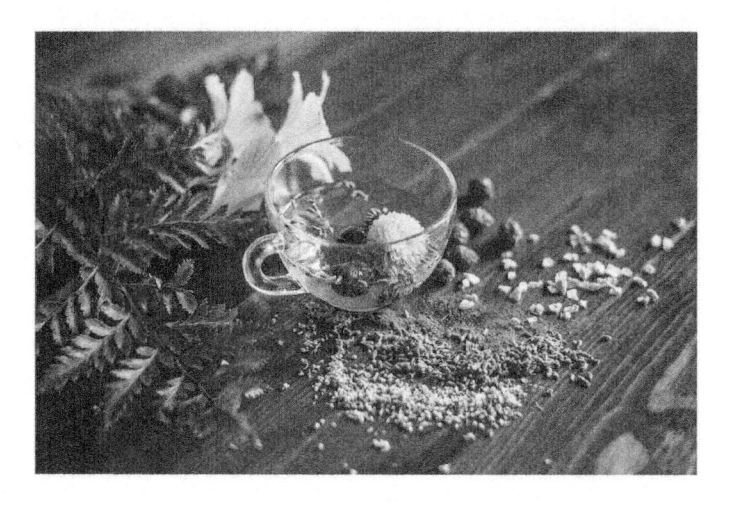

So what can a naturopathic doctor do for a person with NAFLD? There are many options for naturopathic treatment when it comes to liver problems, and a good naturopathic doctor will be happy to review them with you and work out which ones would benefit you most! Just like in traditional medicine, you will be asked to avoid alcohol and sugary drinks like soda as much as possible, and also find a way to lose weight in most cases. Healthy weight management tends to take the form of losing one to two pounds a week through a healthy diet and exercise, while acknowledging that your body needs nourishment and that a starvation diet will only make matters worse! Your naturopathic doctor will also recommend you get the right amount of sleep and exercise, and guide you through finding a routine to do so.

Furthermore, a naturopathic doctor will look into your diet, what changes need to be made, and what nutritional support you might need. This can include taking supplements, such as selenium, probiotics, milk thistle, resveratrol, curcumin, vitamin D, and much more, depending on what you may be deficient in. Finally, naturopathic doctors will figure out what, if any, steps should be taken to cleanse and detoxify harmful chemicals from your system. They may suggest this if you've been exposed to toxins in the environment.

Many naturopathic practitioners make use of herbalism to treat NAFLD and other issues. This is something naturopathy has in common with the other types of whole medicine we'll be discussing here. Herbalism is the practice of using herbs and other plants for their medicinal properties. This is nothing new or unexplored: Herbalism has been used all over the world since the beginning of history, and many over-the-counter or prescription medications include ingredients isolated from plants. Naturopathy draws herbal knowledge from a variety of sources, including TCM and other practices from around the world. One herbal treatment used in naturopathy, TCM, and other whole medicine practices is milk thistle, also called *Silybum marianum* by scientists, which is closely related to daisies! Two extracts from milk thistle, silybin and silymarin, can be included in herbal treatments for NAFLD as they can reduce the effects of inflammation and fibrosis. They can also prevent cells from entering apoptosis, or killing themselves, in response to stress in the liver. A review of herbal treatments for NAFLD by Xiao et al. (2013) revealed that there is actually scientific backing for milk thistle's use to treat fatty liver! In one study, silymarin was tested on two groups of patients, one with NAFLD and one with viral hepatitis. The results showed that silymarin could effectively reduce inflammation from NAFLD thanks to a chemical process not seen in the viral patients (Schrieber et al., 2011).

Traditional Chinese Medicine

Another major form of alternative medicine that can help treat NAFLD is TCM. Forms of TCM have been practiced for thousands of years, and the discipline has developed a rich repertoire of methods to treat a wide range of diseases. TCM approaches the body very differently from mainstream medicine. At the core of TCM is the concept of *qi*, a vital life force that permeates all things. Balancing opposing forces of *yin* and *yang* is also an important part of the practice. TCM practitioners use these concepts to develop treatment plans for all their patients, including people who need help with NAFLD.

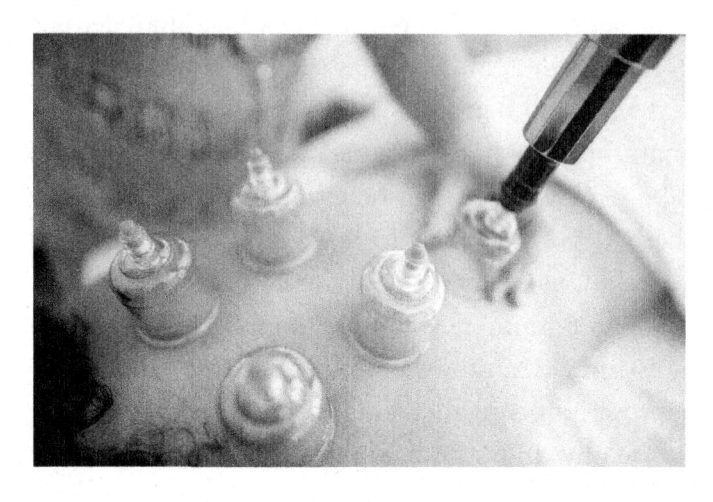

In TCM, the liver plays a range of functions besides the ones acknowledged by mainstream medicine. The liver is closely associated with emotions, as well as with the blood, which is thought to carry *qi* around the body. The TCM method for treating NAFLD is both similar to and different from naturopathy's method. As before, your TCM practitioner will probably ask you about your habits, including diet, sleep, exercise, and vices like drinking and smoking. Just like with naturopathy and even mainstream medicine, lifestyle changes like stepping away from alcohol and eating a healthy diet are integral parts of TCM's approach to NAFLD. However, TCM approaches diet in a bit of a different way. Under TCM, foods belong to different groups depending on their effect on your *qi* as well as your physical body. Eating the right kinds of foods can make your liver stronger and healthier. These include sour foods such as lemon, which TCM teaches are helpful and nourishing to the liver. One TCM practitioner recommends drinking lemon water as part of your liver health routine (Gao, 2017). Lemon is also a diuretic: in other words, it encourages urination. This can help to cleanse unwanted compounds from your body, as many of these are excreted in urine after being cleared from the blood.

In traditional Chinese medicine, ginger supports *yang* and is thought to warm and nourish the blood. TCM practitioners use ginger to settle the stomach and reduce nausea, but also use it to widen blood vessels and encourage decongestion, both very important things to take care of if your liver needs to be detoxed. Since TCM sees the liver as the place where blood is stored and cleansed, taking care of the blood and the liver are intrinsically connected from TCM's point of view. There's also scientific data to back up what ginger can do for your liver under TCM. Ginger can help to reduce inflammation and steatosis, as seen in a recent study examining the effects of ginger supplements on patients with NAFLD (Rahimlou et al., 2016).

Other foods, such as goji berries, are also used to treat liver problems in TCM (Xiao et al., 2013). Also known as wolfberry in English, or by the Chinese name *Gǒu Qǐ Zǐ*, goji berry is a common component in traditional Chinese herbal medicines that target the liver or kidneys. It is also famed for its ability to increase the body's levels of natural antioxidants, which has been demonstrated by serum tests on human volunteers (Xiao et al., 2013). This fascinating berry also activates biochemical pathways associated with the cell's ability to regulate how much fat it carries (Perumpail et al., 2018). Finally, an extensive trial on human volunteers with NAFLD showed that supplementation with goji berries improved all-around outcomes in comparison to the control group. The group that was supplemented with goji berries displayed less fat accumulation in the liver and less inflammation than the control group (Xiao et al., 2013).

Herbalism is just as essential to TCM as it is to other forms of whole medicine, and the discipline has a deep understanding of which kinds of herbs are most useful for treating different health problems. TCM practitioners may recommend you start taking herbs to support your health, based on the traditional Chinese understanding of the effects of each plant. These herbs can be taken in as supplements, or infused into a tea.

One herbal method TCM practitioners use to treat NAFLD is *Lingguizhugan* decoction, sometimes called LGZG for short. The recipe first appears in ancient Chinese literature. According to a recent review by T. Liu et al. (2013), the treatment uses "*Poria (Fulin), Ramulus cinnamomi (Guizhi), Rhizoma atractylodis macrocephalae (Baizhu)*, and *Radix glycyrrhizae (Gancao)*," with the plants' Latin names listed first and their Chinese names in brackets. The decoction works by warming yang and promoting diuresis (Liu, T. et al., 2013), in other words, rebalancing the body's opposing forces and encouraging the body to remove toxins by making it easier to urinate. While scientific trials are still ongoing, this mixture has been used to treat liver issues under the principles of TCM for centuries. Not only that, but the early trials on rats cited by T. Liu et al., showed that the LGZG decoction protected the liver from injury and reduced fat accumulation. Additionally, the LGZG decoction has been used to treat insulin resistance, a risk factor for NAFLD, in humans with some success.

Since the liver is deeply connected to emotion in TCM, looking after your mental and emotional well-being is an important part of treating NAFLD through TCM. It's especially important to manage anger and stress for your liver's health and cleanliness, and TCM practitioners work with their patients to figure out what kind of help is needed in this area. Under TCM, excessive anger and stress are thought to be a sign that the liver may need to be cleansed (Vanbuskirk, 2022).

Finally, your TCM practitioner might recommend you get acupuncture or acupressure therapy. Acupuncture uses electric stimulation with tiny, thin needles inserted in specific points on the body. This is meant to unblock energy paths that may be clogged, in order to allow your body to heal. Acupressure is mostly the same idea except there is no penetration into the skin. Instead, the practitioner applies pressure with fingertips, hands, elbows, toes, or feet to unclog the blockage so the energy can run through. Sometimes the same practitioner will use both acupuncture and acupressure. In the specific case of NAFLD, a particular pressure point in the foot called *taichong* can be manipulated to support your liver and digestive system.

Ayurvedic Medicine

If you're investigating alternative medicine and whole medicine practices, it won't be long until you hear about Ayurveda, also known as

Ayurvedic medicine. The word Ayurveda, which comes from Sanskrit, translates roughly to "knowledge of life" in English. This is a holistic practice that has been around for thousands of years, originating from the Indian subcontinent and cultural beliefs. Ayurveda is a very ancient practice, with the first texts dating back to 3000 BC. At its core, Ayurveda focuses on three *doshas* (*vata, kapha,* and *pitta)*, or vital forces, that exist in different combinations in different individuals. Your unique makeup of *doshas*, or your *prakriti*, determine how your body reacts to everything from stress to food. The practitioner operates with respect to five internal elements (air, fire, water, earth, and space) that are associated with each of the three *doshas* to different degrees. Different organs are linked to these elements, and to the *doshas*, in different ways. The liver is closely connected to fire, as well as *pitta*, which is closely linked to inflammation, digestion, and metabolism, as well as anger, drive, motivation, and ambition. An imbalance of *pitta* and the other *doshas* is thought to lead to liver problems.

When the *doshas* are out of balance, an Ayurvedic practitioner takes steps to realign them. They use dietary and herbal interventions to do this, as well as meditation and other spiritual practices. External application of oils and special massage techniques are also part of this school of medicine. Ayurvedic medicine can be a good choice for anyone who's interested in herbalism, as well as anyone who's open to working on their spiritual as well as their physical health to get their liver back on track.

Just like with other whole medicine practices, an Ayurvedic practitioner will recommend you follow the needed lifestyle changes to combat NAFLD. This includes dietary changes. If your practitioner determines your *pitta* is out of balance, they may recommend you eat bitter, astringent, and sweet-tasting foods to balance it out. On the flip side, they might advise you to stay away from pungent, salty, and sour foods, as these could make the situation worse (*The pitta type in Ayurveda*, n.d.). Ayurvedic medicine also has a number of unique methods for treating NAFLD and other liver problems, which have been in use for hundreds, if not thousands of years. For example, a mixture of traditional herbs can be used to support your liver function, keeping the roles of each of the three *doshas* in mind. Ayurvedic medicines can sometimes contain dozens of herbs (for example, *Pippalyasavam* contains 26!) so don't worry if you need to take some time to research their contents and effects! A good practitioner will also take the time to answer your concerns before you start taking the medicine.

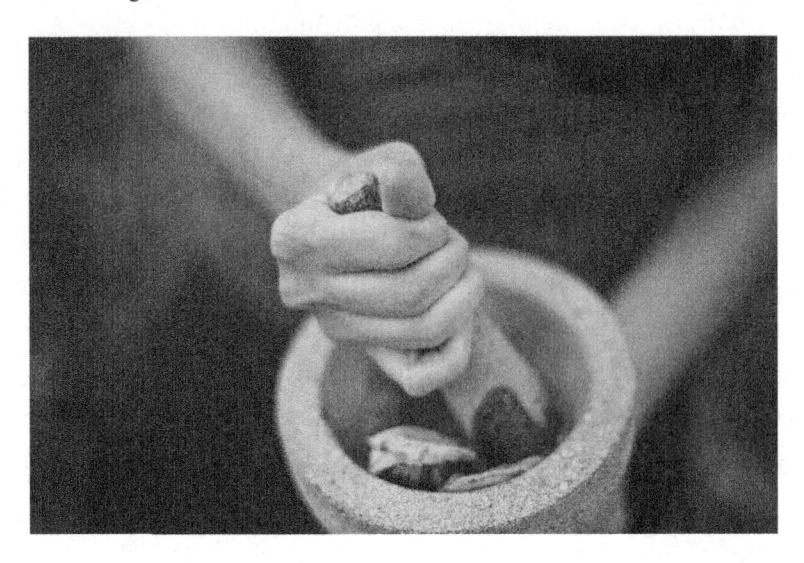

One Ayurvedic medicine that comes up in discussions of NAFLD is *Vasaguduchyadi kashaya*, which is traditionally prepared with 13 ingredients. We don't have space to go through the individual effects of each ingredient, but the medicine includes a special trio of ingredients called *triphala*, which is used alone or mixed into a variety of other Ayurvedic medicines. *Triphala* is made of *amla*, *baheda* and *harad*, all traditional Indian herbs. *Amla* is rich in fiber and antioxidants, making it great for your digestive health. The other two ingredients target liver issues head-on. Along with a range of other uses such as combating diabetes, *baheda* is traditionally used to protect the liver against damage. *Harad* has strong anti-inflammatory effects, helping to reduce the effects of hepatitis while also working to heal the liver. When used in *Vasaguduchyadi kashaya*, the *triphala* herbs are mixed with the other 10 ingredients and either taken as an infusion or as a tablet supplement. Usually, two doses a day are recommended, but be sure to follow your practitioner's instructions if they think another rate would work better for you!

Among the other ways Ayurvedic practitioners treat NAFLD is *Pippalyasavam*, the mixture of 26 traditional herbs we mentioned above. This mixture is used to treat anemia and liver issues, as well as to improve blood circulation and support digestive health. *Amla*, an herb we mentioned in the last paragraph, is also an ingredient in *Pippalyasava*. Another major ingredient is *pippali*, also known as long pepper. In Ayurvedic thought, *pippali* is able to strengthen digestive fire, improve metabolism, and promote healthy blood circulation. It is also thought to make it easier for your body to absorb the other nutrients included in the medicine.

Meditation for Mind and Body

These forms of alternative medicine focus on getting the mind and body working in unison, especially when facing illness and disease. Some of the treatment methods we're going to talk about in this section are used by the forms of alternative medicine we discussed in more detail previously–for example, some Ayurvedic practitioners recommend various forms of meditation to their patients. We split the sections as most of the practices we're about to discuss can also be used to treat NAFLD on their own, regardless of whether you're seeing a naturopathic doctor, TCM practitioner, Ayurvedic medical practitioner, or another alternative school of thought!

The first and foremost of the mind-body therapies we're going to talk about is meditation.

This practice is sometimes associated with specific religions, but people from any faith or cultural background can learn to meditate and reap its benefits. We shouldn't even be talking about meditation as one thing, as there are so many different schools of thought on how to meditate, depending on what your goals are! For example, some forms of meditation require you to sit very still, while others allow you to walk around. Some require you to completely empty your mind, while some include visualization exercises. People meditate for spiritual fulfillment, to help them feel connected to the universe, and to help them cope with daily stressors. This is all great for people who are dealing with a serious illness like NAFLD, as coping skills and spiritual connection can give you both the hope and motivation you need to work on your health. However, the benefits can go much further than that, and as you're about to see, meditation can affect your physical body as well.

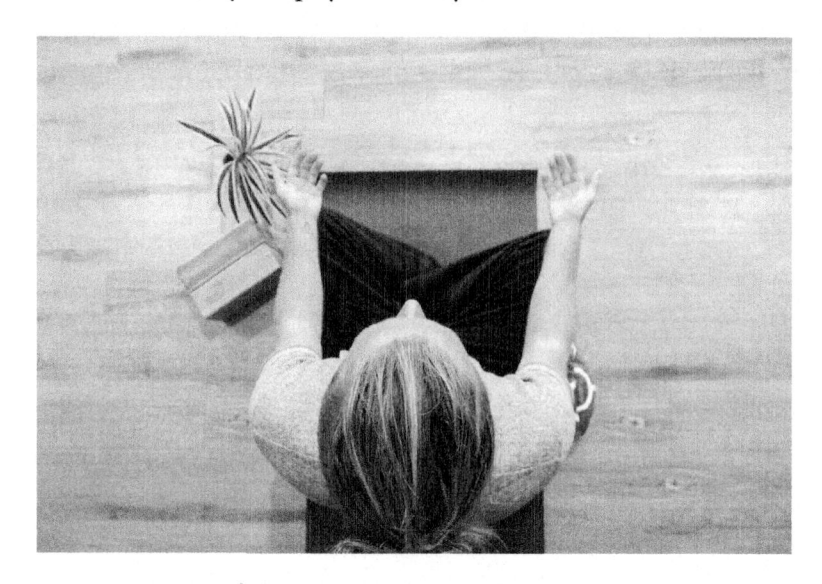

When a holistic practitioner recommends meditation for NAFLD, they may be doing this because meditation can actually reduce the amount of inflammation in your body. Since inflammation is a major part of NAFLD, this can make a difference. There's actual scientific backing to support the idea that meditation fights inflammation, as seen in studies such as the one performed by Creswell et al. (2016) which set out to discover the mechanism behind this phenomenon. That's right– meditation is so well-established as a method to reduce inflammation that Dr. Creswell and his team didn't set out to show that it could, but why that happens!

While they weren't able to explain the entire effect of meditation on inflammation, they showed that meditation forms stronger connections between regions of the brain that, when connected, are associated with a lower risk of inflammatory disease (Creswell et al., 2016). While Creswell and his team didn't set out to explore the connection between meditation and NAFLD specifically, reducing your bodily inflammation is helpful enough that many people include meditation in their NAFLD treatment plans. For example, some holistic doctors and other medical professionals recommend a treatment plan for NAFLD and other inflammatory chronic diseases called mindfulness-based stress reduction (MBSR). MBSR includes meditation as a key component along with other relaxation techniques, exercise, diet, sleep, fostering healthy relationships, mental health counseling, and community engagement like volunteering, and has been shown to be very helpful to people with NAFLD and other chronic illnesses (Merkes, 2010).

Qigoing, Tai Chi, and Yoga

A practice very similar to the type of meditation we just discussed is *qigong*, a Chinese practice involving meditation, breath exercises, and specialized body movements and poses. *Qigong* can improve both your spiritual and physical health, and there is an impressive body of research showing it can be helpful for NAFLD, as it helps manage the effects that excess fat and inflammation have on your body! To start, it's well-established that *qigong* can help reduce the effects of high blood pressure, insulin resistance, and other variables that can increase your risk of or worsen NAFLD. It can also work to help you lose weight (Liu, X. et al., 2008). *Qigong* includes exercises, poses, and routines that are targeted to different organs throughout the body, including the liver, and expert practitioners believe that *qigong* can help improve the flow of blood and energy around the liver and improve its function.

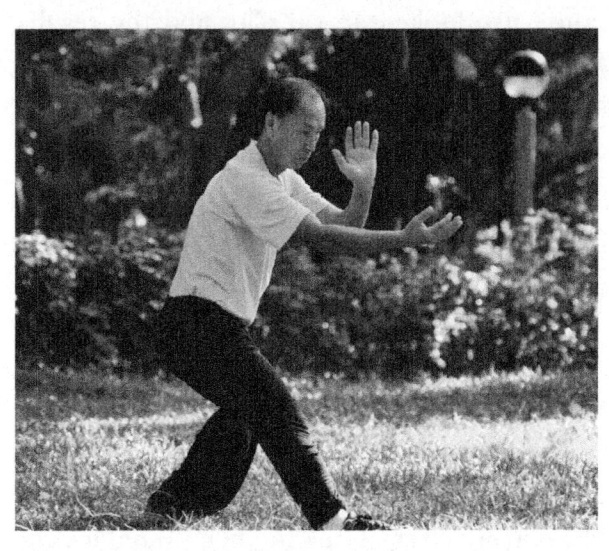

Furthermore, recall that under TCM, the liver is seen as the home of emotions, and that anger, stress, and other negative feelings can affect your liver health. Practicing *qigong* can help you release the emotions, which is healing to your liver in TCM thinking (Liz, 2018). Mainstream medicine is still investigating whether *qigong* can help with NAFLD, but given that it's been shown to help with many related conditions, the odds that it'll be confirmed to work for NAFLD too are promising. While waiting on more data, there's no harm in working *qigong* into your routine: it's great for you anyway, and the evidence we have suggests that it can be very helpful for anyone dealing with an inflammatory illness, including NAFLD.

Similarly, Tai Chi is another ancient Chinese practice that uses slow deliberate movements, poses, and breath control to bring the practitioner into a meditative state. The poses in Tai Chi are often based on martial arts, and the practice is sometimes called shadowboxing as it appears the practitioner is in slow-motion combat with an invisible opponent. Tai Chi and *qigong* are often practiced together, but it's incorrect to conflate them. Like *qigong*, Tai Chi can be helpful for achieving balance and inner peace when coping with life-threatening conditions, including NAFLD, but can also help physically as well. For starters, the same X. Liu et al. (2008) study that demonstrated that *qigong* can help manage blood pressure and insulin resistance also looked at Tai Chi, and the results were just as promising, showing that Tai Chi can help with weight loss and with managing other conditions that can worsen NAFLD. Some expert practitioners of Tai Chi also recommend it for managing NAFLD and other liver conditions, and while mainstream medicine is still investigating its effects in this area, people already report that Tai Chi helped manage their liver issues (Foo, 2018).

If martial arts really aren't your thing, what about looking into yoga instead? Though yoga originated as part of Hinduism, people of any faith or culture can learn the practice. The focus is moving the body slowly through various poses while concentrating on breathing. Yoga not only increases strength and flexibility, it is also an effective way to stretch pain out of muscles, increase circulation, and help to reduce chronic stress. It can also reduce overall bodily inflammation.

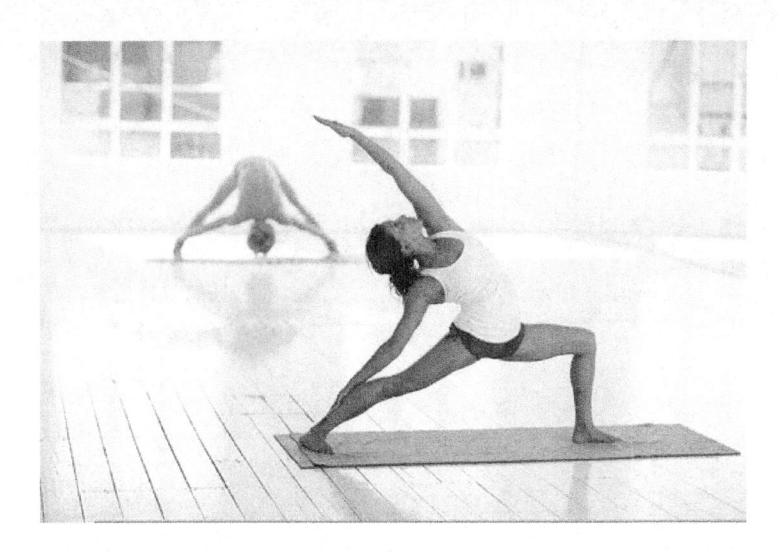

Yoga is commonly recommended as a form of exercise for patients with NAFLD by both alternative and mainstream medical practitioners. If you do some research into the practice of yoga itself, you'll find that there are actual *asanas*, or poses, which are believed to benefit the liver, and which practitioners recommend to people suffering from NAFLD. A few of these are *Padmasana*, the famous "lotus" pose; and *Bhujangasana*, the "cobra" pose where the practitioner lays on their stomach and pushes their chest upwards with their arms. Both of these classic poses, and many more, are thought to stimulate your inner organs and help with NAFLD and similar issues. Don't be afraid to look into lessons or a group class if you think you'd benefit! As great as yoga can be for NAFLD and other liver issues, we need to wrap up this section with a word of caution. Certain poses may cause further injury or damage to the liver, especially when there is inflammation, swelling, or cirrhosis. Be sure to let your coach know about your condition so they can give suggestions on the poses best suited to you, and talk to your doctor before getting started.

PART III

Creating a Liver-Healthy Lifestyle

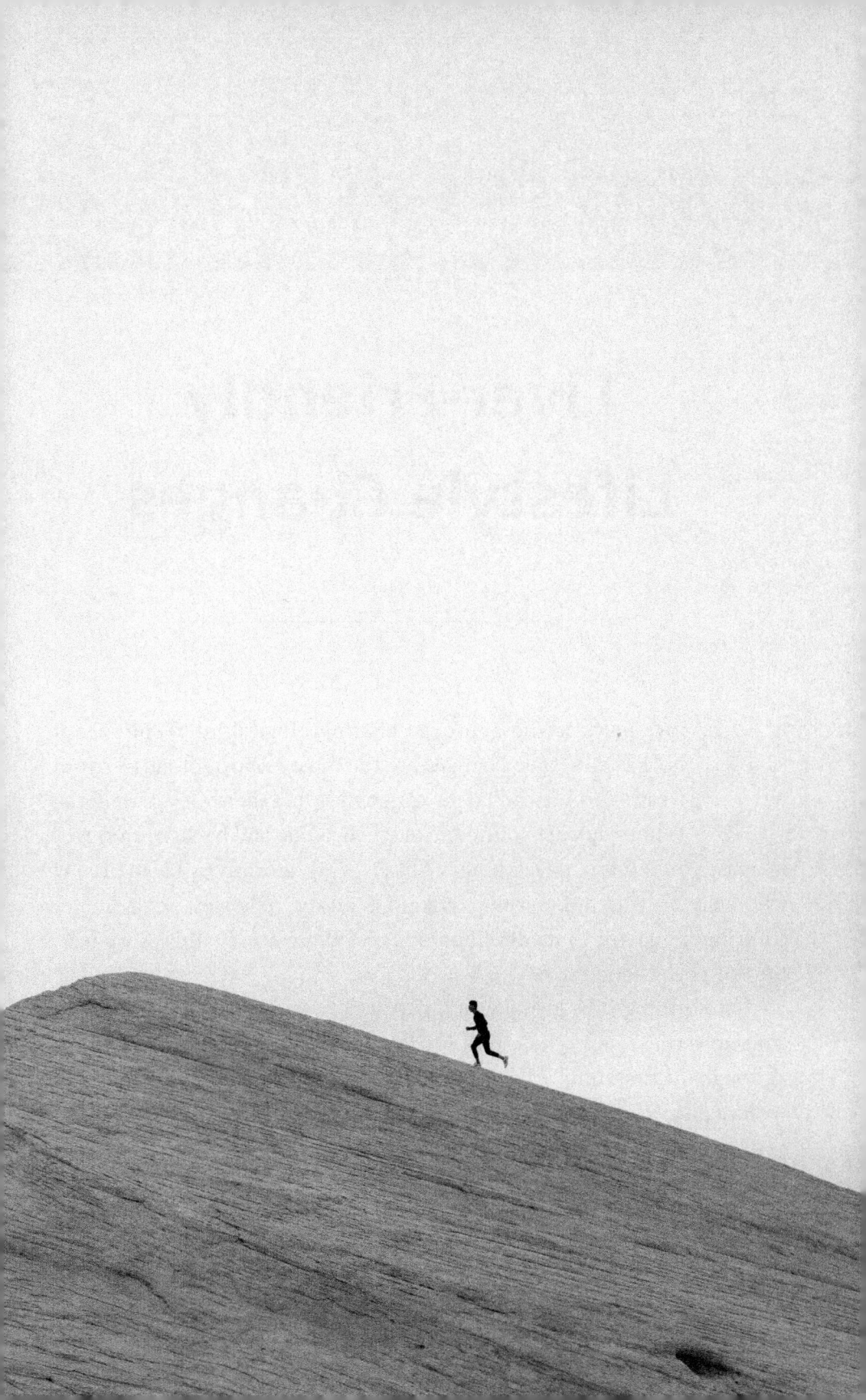

Chapter 5

Liver-Friendly Lifestyle Changes

Since there are no approved pharmacological interventions for NAFLD, lifestyle changes are the most important part of your treatment. We can't control genetics, and there are a number of factors outside your control (such as age and background) that increase your odds of developing NAFLD. While it's impossible to predict who will or will not develop NAFLD, lifestyle choices are a major contributing factor to its development, and those are the things we have the power to change.

Simple things like losing weight, avoiding alcohol, managing diabetes, and lowering your cholesterol will all help with treating NAFLD, although the first thing you'll want to focus on is combining a healthy diet with regular exercise to lose weight. Losing even three to five percent of your overall weight will help you address the circumstances that come from living with NAFLD. Make sure you involve your doctor when it comes to creating a plan for losing weight, ensuring that you are changing your lifestyle by taking small steps that will lead to long-term success. Through simple adjustments to your daily habits, you can take the steps you need to control NAFLD and live a healthier life. We'll also talk about giving up any harmful habits that contribute to your NAFLD, as well as tips on building a more positive mindset to inspire you to keep moving forward. The greatest ally you have is hope, because optimism and motivation are your best friends when it comes to taking control of your health.

How to Build New Habits

Lifestyle changes are the most important aspect of treating NAFLD. These are your best bet when it comes to reversing or managing the condition. One of the most important things to remember when it comes to NAFLD is that the condition probably took a long time to develop, so you won't be able to cure it overnight: reversing the condition will also be a lengthy process. Furthermore, remember that when you're working on making the appropriate lifestyle changes, you have been reinforcing your old, negative habits for years and your positive habits are brand new to you. Therefore, living a healthy lifestyle may not come naturally to you right away. In this section, we've included four helpful tips for forming new, healthy habits that stick and become second nature, allowing you to develop a healthier lifestyle that will last a lifetime. Many of these tips are drawn from the Atomic Habits philosophy, developed by author and expert James Clear (2018).

Start With Small Changes

What you may think of as one habit, may actually be a series of smaller habits that you perform in conjunction. Consider, for example, this negative habit: A person wakes up every morning and spends an hour scrolling through social media in bed before getting up and going about their day. This harms their mental and emotional health through the toxicity that is often present in social media, while also preventing them from having time to exercise in the morning. A pattern like this may increase their stress, especially if they end up being late for work, not to mention they will miss out on all the benefits that exercising regularly has to offer the body and their NAFLD.

There are a number of habits at play here: laying in bed for a long time after the alarm goes off, keeping a smartphone by their bedside, scrolling through social media first thing, and choosing not to exercise in the morning. You'll have more success trying to change habits if you break them down to smaller habits and change them incrementally; instead of fighting against four or five established habits at once, you can try to change them one at a time. In this example, the person could start with resolving to stop keeping their phone at their bedside at night. Perhaps it could be kept at the far side of the room or in a different space entirely to create distance between the habit of scrolling through their phone first thing in the morning. This will also support them getting out of bed sooner since they'll be bored without access to social media. Once they've established leaving their phone in another room as a habit, they can choose the next habit that they'd like to work on, perhaps getting to the gym a few times a week.

When you can focus on making small changes, one at a time, you may find that it's easier to steer your ship in the direction that you'd like it to go. Oftentimes, our mind can feel overwhelmed by change or worried about trying to keep up with everything when we make too much change all at once. If you find yourself in that situation, it's time to take a step back and reevaluate what the biggest motivator will be to help heal your NAFLD. Focus on that, and only that, for two to three weeks until it becomes second nature before you add in something else.

Connect New Habits to Current Habits

Since the habits you have currently are well-established in your brain, it can be helpful to use this to your advantage as you work to change them one by one. Our minds enjoy routine, familiarity, and comfort, so when you can tweak old habits that you enjoy, instead of working to eliminate them entirely, you may find that there's less resistance to making that change happen. For example, let's go back to the idea of a person who skips exercising in the morning because they spend a lot of time scrolling on their phone. This person could resolve to only look through their favorite social media sites if they're walking on the treadmill. This will encourage them to stick to the new habit (exercising) by connecting it to an old habit (social media). If this person later decides to reduce the amount of time they spend on social media, they can find a healthier form of entertainment to consume during their treadmill time instead. By bridging the two together, the habit of exercising becomes much easier to follow through on and doesn't require restricting an enjoyable activity in order to be successful.

Give Yourself Something to Look Forward to

Sometimes building new habits can start with giving yourself something to look forward to that is attached to the healthier choice. This doesn't mean to reward yourself by engaging in unhealthy habits after you manage to stick to healthy ones, but to do whatever you can to make the new habit appealing and pleasurable. There are many ways to build discipline, but you may find it helpful to use rewards at the end of a task to reinforce the habit. A great way to stay consistent enough to transition over from feeling like you're working hard to stick with a new habit and changing it into a second nature behavior, is by building in small things that you look forward to having or doing, either during or after practicing your new habit.

For example, the person who is trying to replace their daily social media consumption with time at the gym might make themselves a special playlist to listen to while they work out, or download an interesting podcast to listen to. They may spend time creating a variety of music choices depending on the type of exercise, or certain podcasts for different days, but in order to listen they must follow through on their exercise plan. The key here is to only engage in the reward activity while doing the habit you want to establish. By associating something fun with your new habit, it won't be long for your brain to learn that if it wants that particular pleasurable experience or treat, you need to follow through.

Get Back on the Horse

If you slip up and have a bad day where you fall back into old habits, it doesn't have to be the end of the world. Look at backslides as a learning experience and use them to avoid making the same mistakes again in the future. You will have days where life has thrown what feels like a million curveballs at you, and you won't make it to the gym or eat in the perfect way you should. That's okay—you are human and making choices, choices that aren't the best for you, happens to all of us. The best thing to do when you fall off track is to forgive yourself, remember your reason for wanting to reach your goal and follow through on your new habits, and then let that moment be the time you start afresh. The minute you realize that you've gone down a slippery slope, is the exact moment you can hit refresh and start making different choices. For example, if the person in our hypothetical scenario finds themselves scrolling through their phone in the gym locker room instead of starting their workout, they'll know they have to find a way to avoid that in the future. They could use parental controls or the Guided Access setting to block access to social media from their phone except for during specific times of day, or they could turn off their phone and leave it in the bottom of their bag, safe and sound in their locker.

Most importantly, it's essential for them to become creative with building separation between the bad habit that is stopping them from taking action and pursuing their new ones. Part of habit building is knowing that you cannot give up and must keep pushing towards the goals you've set for yourself, despite any setbacks you might encounter. The example of the person who doesn't have time to exercise or shortens their dedicated workout time because of scrolling through social media is just a theoretical one, but you can apply the philosophy we've described above to any habit in your life. By setting realistic goals, making small changes, and using the way your brain solidifies habits to your advantage, you can give yourself the best possible odds of making the lifestyle changes you need to make.

Upgrading Your Mindset

When you are diagnosed with NAFLD or any other serious condition, you may be feeling a mix of emotions, including fear, regret, stress, and anger. You might feel inclined to think negatively of yourself and your choices, to worry about the future, or to dread making the necessary changes you need to improve your health. While many people scoff at the idea that a positive or negative attitude can affect your physical health, both holistic and traditional medicine are well aware of this fact. In fact, multiple studies on the effect of a positive outlook on health outcomes back up the idea that people who are optimistic are healthier in the long run (Harvard Health Publishing, 2019). Furthermore, according to the beliefs that underpin TCM and some other alternative medicine practices, the liver is deeply connected to your emotional state. In this section, we've included five helpful tips for improving your mindset, in order to improve your liver health and your health as a whole.

Keep Track of Stressors

One of the main reasons people have trouble staying positive is that they're dealing with chronic stress. Chronic stress can feel overwhelming and can increase inflammation levels in the body, which may worsen the symptoms of NAFLD. One project you can do when you want to start turning around your mindset is to start carrying a small notebook or journal with you, and writing down things and situations that make you feel unhappy or stressed. Then at the end of every word or sentence write the phrase, "This too I can handle" or "This will get better". Having them all written down in front of you can make them seem much more manageable, and reading the affirmation at the end can help change the way your mind approaches or feels about that particular pain point. You can also do this in the Notes app of your smartphone if you don't have access to a physical pen and paper.

Remember the Good in Life

When stress and other negative life situations are piling up, it can be hard to think of the things that make you happy and you may find that your mind fixates on what you are worrying about. However, remembering that there are fun and positive aspects to life is essential to cultivating a positive mindset. This is another area where journaling what you are grateful for in the morning or evening can be really helpful or practicing gratitude by simply saying out loud, in the moment, "I am grateful for (fill in the blank)". For example, you can write down anything that makes you smile, things that you look forward to, or just anything that happens that you'd like to remember in a positive way, including the fact that you are working to improve your NAFLD symptoms and prognosis. Having a list of the positive aspects of your life laid out in front of you will help you remember the good and can be helpful for picking yourself up when you're feeling down.

Spend Time With Friends and Loved Ones

If you are feeling very down or sad much of the time, you might be feeling socially isolated. The COVID-19 pandemic has been a stark reminder of how important it is to socialize for the sake of your mental health. While it can be hard to spend a lot of time with people who make you happy, such as friends and family, when you're busy and stressed, try to make time for it at least a few times a week. This is one area where the internet can be very helpful, though most people find in-person social interactions the most beneficial. Support groups can be found online or even in-person near your home, and are typically free to attend. Use a simple internet search to find one that you can attend to stay connected with people and re-engage with the world. At the same time, try to avoid negative and toxic people as much as you can, since these individuals can bring your mood down more than you may realize.

Learn to Manage Stress

As we've mentioned above, stress can be a major reason why you're having trouble staying positive. It can also be very harmful to your body by increasing blood pressure, making it harder to sleep, and affecting the hormones and liver enzymes in your bloodstream. Therefore, learning to manage stress is essential to improving your physical and mental health, and to adopting a positive mindset. Most people forget that they need to manage their stress on a daily basis, just like drinking water or getting enough sleep. Healthy mental hygiene comes from identifying stress in your life and taking practical steps to release your anxieties, fears, and worries surrounding it. You'll know if your body feels stressed by how tight your muscles feel, how stiff parts of your body are, or how achy you may feel that day.

The previous chapter discussed a number of practices that incorporate physical, spiritual, and mental aspects of health in order to help you learn to cope with stress, such as meditation, pranayama, yoga, Tai Chi, and pilates. Learning to practice one or more of these on a daily basis will provide you with valuable tools to improve your mindset overall. Getting some exercise, practicing your religious or spiritual beliefs, and spending time in nature can also be valuable ways to cope with stress. You deserve to do the little things that bring you joy and peace every single day.

Seek Help if Needed

If you follow all these steps and you still feel sad, down, or negative most of the time, there might be a mental health condition such as depression at play. There's no shame in seeking help for your mental health: Billions of people around the world struggle with mental health conditions every day! Talking to a therapist or to your primary doctor can get you on the road to evaluating whether you're struggling with a mental health problem, and what avenues are available to help you overcome it. Depending on your therapist, your doctor, and your personal situation, you may be prescribed medication, be recommended to start talk therapy, or be referred to a specialist.

Weight Loss

Unless you are underweight or malnourished, your primary physician is likely going to recommend that you lose weight as a part of your treatment plan. Depending on their school of thought and your personal situation, you may be asked to lose between three and five percent of your total body weight for the health of your liver. While weight loss can seem daunting, especially if you've struggled to lose weight in the past, it's not impossible if you have patience and discipline. Remember that you didn't get to your current weight overnight, so you won't get down to a healthy weight overnight either! Here, we've included three essential tips for losing weight in a healthy manner.

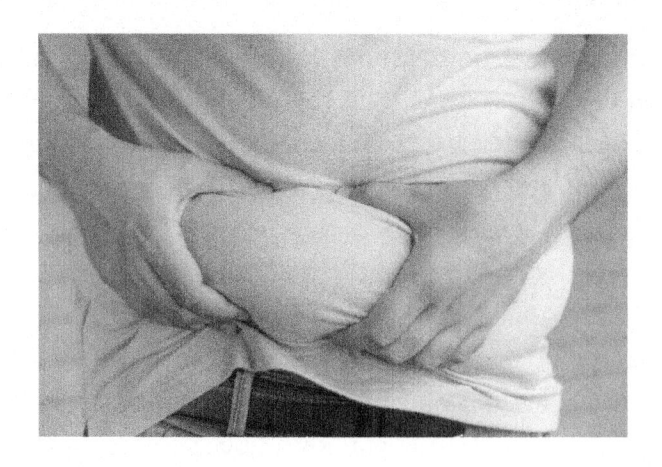

Eat Intuitively

This doesn't mean to give in to every craving for sweet and salty snacks, but to pay attention to your body's hunger and satiety signals. Eating intuitively means eating only when you're hungry–this means properly hungry with a growling stomach, not just feeling like you could eat. It also means stopping, not when you've finished your plate, but when your hunger is satisfied. Learning to eat intuitively can reduce the need for calorie counting or similar measures, as you'll only be taking in what your body needs.

Intuitive eating is not for everyone. Certain people who struggle with obesity may have resistance to the hormones our body uses to tell us when we're satisfied, putting them at risk for overeating. Talk to your doctor to determine whether you deal with this kind of issue. If you aren't confident in your ability to eat intuitively, consider counting calories or using a program like Weight Watchers to keep track of how much you're taking in.

Avoid Snacking

When trying to lose weight, remember that you don't need to be feeling full every second of the day. Eating a lot of snacks adds up quickly, and the foods people commonly snack on are often full of fructose, saturated fats, sodium, and other addictive compounds that are terrible for your liver. On top of eating intuitively, try your best to avoid snacking in between meals by applying the habit-forming tips we discussed earlier in this chapter. If you must snack, opt for raw, unsalted nuts and seeds instead of candy, as these are satisfying, great for your liver health, and packed with healthy fats and fiber.

Choose Healthy Fats

Your body needs fats to function, even when you're dealing with NAFLD or another form of fatty liver disease. However, not all fats are good for you. Recall how we've previously defined the difference between unhealthy saturated and healthy unsaturated fats, and how unsaturated fats can be good for the health of your liver. Unsaturated fats are also great at triggering the secretion of satiety hormones such as leptin, which are your body's mechanism for telling you that you've had enough to eat. This will make it easier to avoid snacking between meals, and to eat smaller portions at your regular eating times.

Exercise

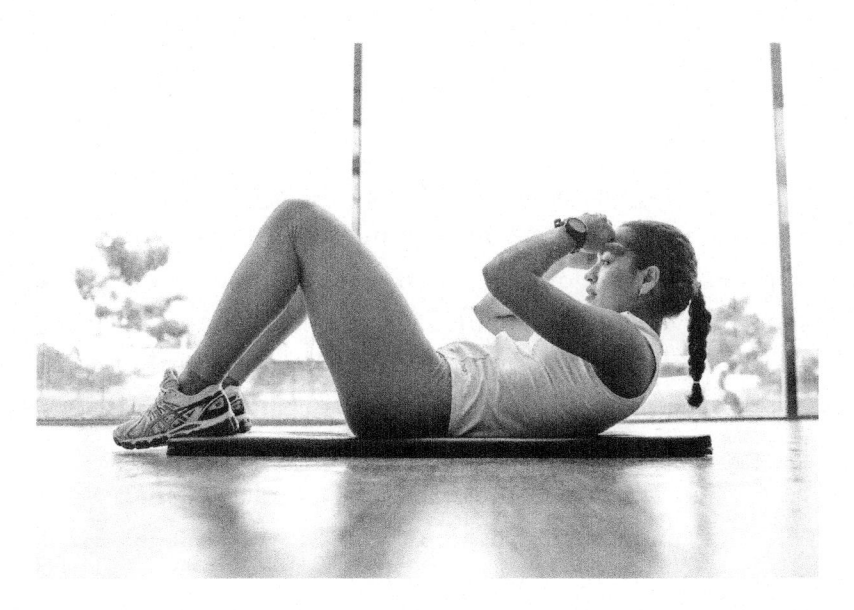

Exercise is one of the most important aspects of healthy weight loss, and your doctor may recommend that you exercise regardless of whether you lose weight. Exercise encourages your body to metabolize stored energy, including fat, which can help fight the buildup of excess fat in the liver. Exercise will also reduce how much fat your liver synthesizes, as this energy is needed to support the vigorous activity you're doing. It also burns calories, since it takes more energy to exercise than to be sedentary.

It can also increase your appetite for healthy foods, making it much easier to stick to your liver-friendly diet. Many forms of exercise can help you build muscle to replace the fat you lose, which is an important part of losing weight in a healthy manner. Finally, exercise is commonly recommended to people who are trying to quit unhealthy habits such as drinking, smoking, or drugs, as exercise can help relieve the stress and cravings that cause people to engage in these habits.

There are a number of types of exercise that can be beneficial to your weight-loss goals. We've explored a few of them in a bit more detail here. Furthermore, most practitioners would agree that both cardio (or aerobic) exercise and strength exercise are beneficial to people suffering from NAFLD and NASH (Fatty Liver Disease, 2021). With the help of your doctor and the rest of your medical team, you can develop an exercise plan that is not only healthy for your liver, but also suits your health goals overall.

Cardio Training

The first of the major forms of exercise is cardio, which revolves around raising your heart rate for a period of time before bringing it back down. This is done by doing some form of continuous physical activity using the power of your own body. Running, swimming, rowing, boxing, and cycling are all sports that rely heavily on cardio. Furthermore, team sports like soccer, football, basketball, and baseball all require a high level of ability in cardio, and cardio exercises are a major part of training for these sports. Cardio is great for people who have followed their physician's advice to stop smoking after being diagnosed with liver disease; cardio helps repair existing lung damage, as it encourages the lungs to regenerate in order to accommodate the additional work they have to do.

Cardio exercises usually take place over a period of 10 minutes at a minimum, and can continue up to several hours. Not only does this burn a lot of fat, especially if your heart rate reaches a high level, but it also improves the capacity of your cardiovascular system, helping to manage many of the diseases that are comorbid with being obese or overweight.

For example, cardio is a great way to reduce the amount of triglycerides in your bloodstream, lowering your risk of both NAFLD and heart disease. Furthermore, cardio is a great way to boost your daily energy levels, which can make it much easier to stick to the healthy lifestyle habits you've been working on.

Many cardio athletes rave about loading up on carbs before their cardio workouts in order to give themselves a boost of energy before they get going. While it's true that your body can really benefit from carbs when it's going to be doing a cardio workout, remember that it's healthiest for your liver to avoid sugar and refined carbs as much as possible (we'll be talking more about this in the following chapter). Foods with refined carbs include white bread and white pasta, both of which are popular with cardio athletes. Instead of loading up on carbs, opt for a varied diet of whole grains, vegetables, lean proteins, and healthy fats in order to give yourself the nutrition you need to get through your workouts.

Beans and brown rice with baked chicken breast and a side salad, for example, makes a great, liver-healthy meal for a cardio athlete. Oatmeal is also very liver-healthy while containing the carbs you need to keep working out. Furthermore, be sure that you drink plenty of water and replace electrolytes when you're working out in this manner, as these make all the difference to how much energy you have. Electrolytes are small, electrically charged molecules that play an important role in your muscle function, and having too little will result in fatigue. They can be replaced by drinking bone broth or a sports drink such as Gatorade (remember to opt for a low-sugar version of the beverage if you go this route!)

Finally, a few safety concerns should be noted. Pay attention to your body when you do cardio. If you feel like you've injured yourself, don't try to push through the workout or you may make it much worse. Furthermore, if you feel dizzy, nauseous, and lightheaded, stop the workout immediately and have some water and food. This could be a sign of low blood sugar, which could lead to fainting and falls if you try to push through it.

Strength and Resistance Training

Another popular type of exercise is strength training, which uses weight or resistance to improve the strength of your skeletal muscle. Strength training is also great for burning fat, as it takes a lot of energy to lift heavy weights. While weightlifting is one of the most popular ways to engage in strength training, you can also use resistance bands, exercise machines, weighted medicine balls, and even your own body weight when working out to provide the resistance you need. Strength training is important to practitioners of all martial arts, as well as people who play contact sports like football and rugby. Rowers, climbers, and boulderers can also use strength training to improve their performance.

Strength training works by breaking down your muscles over the course of the workout. The muscles are then repaired during the rest period between workouts, making them stronger than they were before. For this reason, resting in between strength workouts is something you absolutely cannot skip. The great thing about strength training is that you can perform lifts that only engage certain muscle groups, allowing you to work out some muscle groups on the days other ones are resting.

Strength training relies heavily on anaerobic respiration, which is your body's process for creating energy when oxygen is in limited supply. This occurs when you're lifting very heavy weights. The enzyme that facilitates this process, L-lactate dehydrogenase, produces lactic acid as a byproduct, hence the burning feeling you get in your muscles during a workout. The most important aspect of strength training is to try and lift more and more as time goes on, to improve your anaerobic capacity as well as your muscle strength. Anaerobic respiration relies on glycogen stored in the muscles, so it's essential that you don't completely cut carbs from your diet when you're strength training. By using up its glycogen stores, we encourage the liver to burn fat which helps restore it to a healthy state. As with cardio, a balanced diet of whole grains, healthy fats, lean proteins, and vegetables is the best way to go to support strength training and muscle growth.

As a safety measure, start every lift with low weight or only the bar before doing it with weight so you can practice the movement and develop correct form. Furthermore, ensure that you have a realistic view of your abilities and are setting realistic lifting goals. Having the right form and being steady with your movements is more important and beneficial than lifting heavy and not doing it correctly. If you find yourself in a gym or working out with a friend, you can ask them to spot you for any heavy lifts that you want to practice. It will help you avoid dropping weights and getting injured as a result.

Exercising Every Day

You don't have to go to the gym to exercise. Going for a jog, bicycle ride, swim, walk, or hike are all valid ways to get your blood pumping and help with your weight-loss goals. These methods have the added advantage of potentially getting you outdoors in nature, as well as being great activities to do with a friend or partner! Furthermore, if you're resting up from a more structured kind of exercise, this kind of active fun can allow you to keep breaking a sweat, even on your day off. However, don't force yourself to exercise if you're so sore from other types of training that it's painful, or if your doctor has limited how many days a week you need to be exercising!

Bodyweight exercises are any exercises that require no equipment, and use the weight of your own body to provide resistance. There are ways to work bodyweight strength and cardio exercises into your daily routine in a manner that takes very little time out of your day. In other words, time isn't really an excuse when it comes to working out! For example, one common practice is to designate a specific door in your home, and do a bodyweight exercise every time you walk through it. This works best if it's a door you use often and can't avoid going through periodically, like the door to the kitchen or bathroom. Set a goal, such as doing five pushups or squats every time you enter or leave the kitchen, and stick to it as much as possible. Tying a ribbon around the door handle or across the doorway can serve to remind you of your goal. Once your upper body strength improves, you can even look into installing a pull-up bar in one of your home's doorways!

Another way to work exercise into your daily routine is to set a timer for every 30-40 minutes of your work day, and take a short exercise break whenever it goes off. This could take the form of a few bodyweight exercises, a short brisk walk, or some yoga stretches, before getting back to work. This also serves to get your blood moving during the day and prevent stiffness and discomfort from sitting.

Finally, look for ways to make your daily routine more physically active. Options for this include taking the stairs instead of the elevator, walking short distances instead of driving, engaging in active play with your children, and standing instead of sitting whenever you can. It's essential to talk to your doctor before starting any new exercise routine, especially if you have health concerns such as NAFLD. Not every type of exercise is appropriate for every person. Your doctor can advise you on how to exercise safely in order to get the maximum benefit possible for your liver and your overall health.

PART IV

Healing Fatty Liver Through Diet

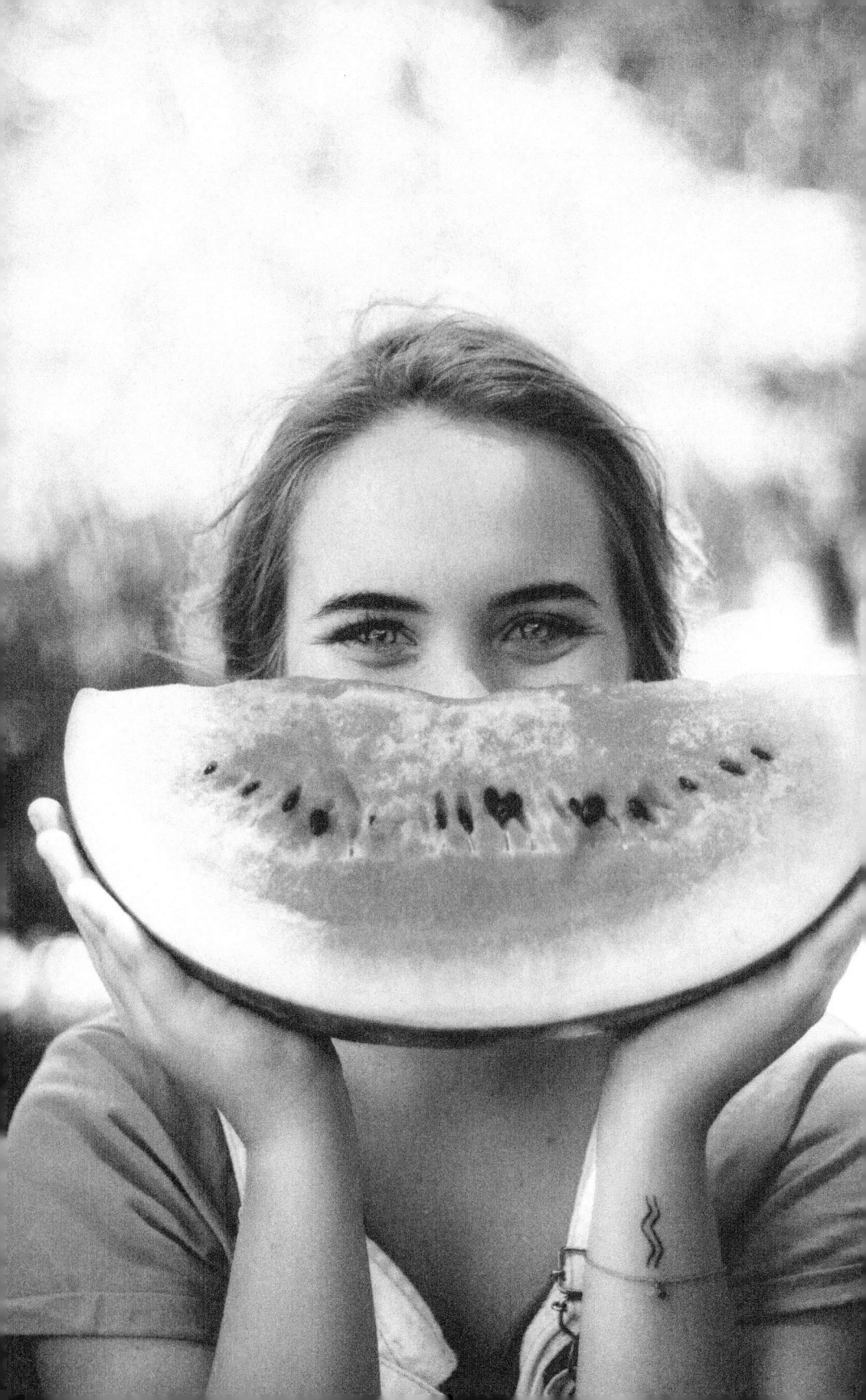

Chapter 6

Creating Your Fatty-Liver Diet Plan

In this section, we're going to put everything together by creating a fatty-liver diet that is best-suited to what your liver needs most. Before moving any further, it's vital that you prioritize your doctor's insights and suggestions. What may work great for one individual may not for another or may make someone's situation worse. For many people, the word diet alone elicits negativity. Diets can be seen as restrictive, rigid, and a lot of work. However, in order to reverse fatty liver disease, eating a healthy diet will become your go-to lifestyle. In the beginning, it may seem like an overwhelming or time-consuming process, but in the end it will be worth it. With time, your body's preferred dietary choices will become second nature and you'll find that with some research and creativity, you can create delicious, interesting recipes that you can enjoy.

That being said, although science has outlined the essentials of foods that are helpful or harmful to your liver, your specific diet plan will be unique to you and your needs. In this chapter, we'll go into more detail about how to create the right diet for your needs, which foods you'll want to include in your plan, common foods that you'll need to avoid, and why all of these instructions will work in your favor. You will be fully equipped to build the right diet for what your liver needs to slow down, heal, and even reverse any damage that has been done. After all, the better you take care of your liver, the better it can take care of you.

Lifestyle and Diet Changes

It may be helpful for you to not think of your diet adjustments as restrictions, but rather small, ongoing lifestyle changes. Being thoughtful about the food you are consuming on a daily basis and choosing to eat or not to eat something will now be a part of your lifestyle. Rather than see a long list of types of foods or dishes that are not good for you, look at how it will affect your body. Will it have a positive or negative impact? What will the food do for your weight, energy levels, emotional support, and liver health? If you find yourself tempted to eat something you know you shouldn't, think about the future effects it will have and how it will work against all the other work you're doing to heal or reverse your liver damage.

Besides, there are thousands of delicious dishes you can incorporate into your nutritional plan; you only have to be willing to explore new cultures, ways of cooking, and tweak what you order when going out to restaurants or eating take out. A common recommendation by doctors is to follow a Mediterranean style of diet. This includes things like olive oil for healthy fats, eating plant-based foods or dishes, and increasing the amount of fruits, vegetables, whole grains, nuts, and lean cuts of meat that you eat. It's what you would expect to hear from any nutritionist, doctor, or dietician—reduce foods that are high in sugars, avoid processed foods, and eat more things in a natural state. If you don't enjoy cooking or preparing meals, you can always purchase vegetables and lean cuts of meat in their frozen state and combine them together in the oven or microwave, adding spices or sauces that match the Mediterranean diet plan for more flavor.

The Mediterranean diet has a wide variety of dishes and flavor combinations you can try in your diet, emphasizing fruits, vegetables, whole grains, and nuts partnered with lean meats like poultry, eggs, seafood, and fish every week. While it may feel hard in the beginning to adapt to this new way of eating, remember that this will be worth it in the long run. Try to avoid the convenience of fast-food or highly processed options by planning in advance to bring food with you, say to work, or to cook a large meal when you are less pressed for time that you can eat over several days. By simplifying how often you spend time cooking, you may find that it's simpler to stick with your meal plans because the convenience will be built in.

You can use one ingredient several different ways to add variety to your meals. This will reduce the risk of feeling bored with what you're eating and seeking out foods that would irritate your liver and send all your hard work backwards. For example, you could cook four to six servings of whole grain rice or quinoa and use that as a base for all your meals that week. When adding lean meats like chicken or fish, you can cook two at a time and then rotate which is eaten for lunch or dinner in either a salad, wrap, or family-style meal. This same strategy works for vegetables, as they'll typically keep for the next day, and can be added to your morning breakfast scramble or warmed back up for dinner. For things like avocados or softer vegetables like tomatoes, try to only cut those the day of, to avoid spoiling or a soggy texture that doesn't taste good with your meal.

Remember, you can also prepare and cook in large batches things like soups or stews because they store well and offer a larger variety of ways to combine foods and flavors to create an interesting diet. Experiment with new spices and ways to cook things, using your oven, a pan, and a grill if you have one to change the flavor profile of what would normally be a vegetable or cut of meat that you don't enjoy. Changing how you season, prepare, and cook a dish will make a large difference in whether or not you find something that tastes good and has umami. Eating healthy and following a diet plan that will help heal your liver will not be boring when you view this change as an opportunity to explore new flavors, dishes, and ways of eating that you'd otherwise never be exposed to. It may surprise you how much you can actually enjoy following your nutrition plan, and not feel restricted from processed, sugary, or fatty foods. Over time, your taste buds and body will adjust to your new way of eating and you'll find that your cravings for unhealthy foods will decrease because you're getting everything you need in your existing diet.

Changing Your Daily Calories

Maintaining a healthy weight or even losing weight will be one of your top priorities when working to manage and heal NAFLD. Weight loss has been shown to decrease the fat in your liver. A simple way to promote weight loss is to reevaluate how many calories you are eating in a day, and where those calories are coming from. If you are unsure of how many calories in a day you are eating, try keeping a food diary for a week or two, writing down what you eat and drink and the corresponding calorie count. You can use food apps on your phone to calculate calories or you can look up the number with an internet search. A good rule of thumb is to reduce your calorie count by 500-1,000 calories to see weight loss results. However, as with everything else we've discussed, make sure that you are not decreasing your calorie intake too much and putting yourself at risk for being malnourished. Talk with your doctor about changing your calorie intake and what the appropriate reduction would be based on your body mass.

When you are reducing how many calories you eat in a day, it's common to feel hungry or sluggish at the beginning until your body adjusts. A great strategy to combat this and avoid binging on foods you are working to keep away from, is to eat smaller meals more frequently throughout the day. Instead of three large meals, try six or seven small portions. These can be healthy snacks like nuts and berries or they can be complete meals just in smaller portions. Learning the right portions for your body and how to stay in a healthy range will help you keep within your recommended calorie count for weight loss. More often than not, we are served double or triple portions of what we should be eating and this has become our expected amount of food. Switch out the plates you use to smaller ones so your food looks visually big, or double up on your vegetables so it takes up most of the space on a large plate. The goal is to not to be hungry or feel like you aren't eating enough, but to slowly adjust how much you're eating without your mind feeling like it's missing out on something fun that it wants.

Try slowing down when you are eating so your mind has time to wait for the stomach to signal that it is full. Feeling satiated takes about twenty minutes from the time you start eating; if you are finishing your meals in two to four minutes, your body has never had a chance to know if it feels full yet and will seek out more food, putting you off your calorie count goals for the day. Work on slowing down and eating with the purpose of enjoying your meal. You can help this along by cutting things into smaller bites, placing your utensils down in between chewing, drinking water in between eating, and timing yourself with a stopwatch to bring awareness to how quickly you've been consuming your meals. Obviously smaller snacks like a handful of nuts won't take 20 minutes to complete, but the intention of slowing down and allowing yourself to feel full still remains, no matter the size of the meal you're eating at that moment.

Supplements That Help Your Liver

Unhealthy eating such as saturated fats, trans fats, simple sugars, and animal protein will build up your overall fat in the body, reduce your sensitivity to insulin, create an imbalance in your gut, and slow down your liver's ability to synthesize fatty acids, which is necessary for the cells in our body to function correctly. Eating vegetable proteins, fiber, and probiotics all support your liver with their antioxidant properties. They promote insulin sensitivity, boost the body's immunity, and prevent any intestinal bacteria that creates disease from invading your tissues and organs. Things like simple sugars, saturated and trans fats, and animal proteins will increase the amount of sodium, additives, and preservatives in your body and cause your liver to work under higher stress, experience dysfunction at a cellular level, and be susceptible to diseases (Perdomo et al., 2019). Essentially, these types of foods throw your liver completely off its tracks and into a wilderness filled with problems.

Since your gut health is related to the functionality of your liver, you'll want to make sure your diet contains prebiotic fiber. This can be found in foods like asparagus, leeks, onions, and garlic. Prebiotics support your gut's health by fermenting nondigestible food, establishing a balanced environment to digest what you eat. Ensuring that you are ingesting enough prebiotic fiber, either through naturally-occurring foods or supplements, will help you with weight loss; your internal organs and digestive system will work more efficiently and you'll feel better as a whole. Including prebiotics will reduce the amount of fat your liver is holding onto, decrease inflammation in the liver's lobes, and stop liver cell degeneration, also called ballooning. There was a pilot trial that supported these findings in patients after 24 weeks of the prebiotic fructooligosaccharide and the probiotic *Bifidobacterium longum*. Combined together, they worked to stimulate weight loss, reduce inflammation, and heal the liver (Lambert et al., 2015).

Fructooligosaccharides are used as an alternative to sugary sweeteners and can be found naturally occurring in foods like bananas, onions, artichokes, garlic, asparagus, yacon root, blue agave, and chicory. They can also be found in syrups, like yacon root and blue agave, that you can dilute in water and take as a supplement. A simple way to include them in your diet is to incorporate those foods into your daily or weekly meals. You could also switch out your sugar in your tea, coffee, or healthy baked goods with this alternative. *Bifidobacterium longum* can be found in foods like yogurt, sauerkraut, and kimchi—dairy items and vegetables that are fermented. It can survive tough conditions in your gut such as stomach acid or changes in your body's pH, and attaches itself to the lining of your intestines. Its tenacity and ability to help digestion make it a great probiotic option. You can find it in supplemental form if you do not enjoy or are unable to eat fermented dairy products or vegetables. Be sure to eat both these in moderation and as a part of a wide, varied diet so as to avoid potential imbalance or overuse.

While you should already be receiving all your vitamins and minerals in a natural way from your diet, it could be that you may need supplemental help to get your levels to a healthy number. One of the more important vitamins, vitamin E, can be readily found in a balanced Mediterranean-style diet, and helps your liver heal by breaking down antioxidants in the body. You don't want to live with the side effects of any vitamin deficiency, especially when certain ones will support your mission to reverse the effects of NAFLD and NASH. A study showed that taking daily vitamin D supplements decreased patients' insulin resistance and had a positive effect on their cardiovascular system as well (Cicero et al., 2018). You can get your vitamin D from foods like salmon, tuna, and fortified dairy and juices, while adding in almonds, red bell peppers, peanuts, collard greens, and spinach will help with your vitamin E. Eating natural, readily available foods will help you incorporate these essential vitamins into your meals, but you can also supplement your dosage by taking these vitamins and others on a daily basis with or without your food.

By sticking with eating more of a Mediterranean, plant-focused diet, and including a variety of liver-healthy supplements, you can reduce the amount of stress your liver is under and support its health, bringing back balance and homeostasis among your internal organs. Our food isn't just what we eat, it's how we fuel and nourish our body. If you are eating meals and types of foods that are difficult for your body to process, such as things high in salt, sugar, or chemicals, it will struggle and eventually be limited in how effective it can work. The body was not made to live on a high-sugar, processed diet, so it makes sense that prolonged exposure to breaking down and absorbing these kinds of foods would wear on it. Take the approach of changing your diet to be focused on helping your body and liver recover so it can regain its full potential and efficiency; you may find that incorporating these new habits isn't as challenging as it initially felt like it would be.

Your Liver-Healthy Diet: Foods to Include

The first step in developing your diet plan is to take a close look at the foods you're putting into your body right now. An important note here is that many foods we choose to eat may not be the problem on their own. How foods are prepared also matters. The simplest example is a potato, which is high in both potassium and antioxidants that the liver needs. If that potato is drizzled with olive oil, seasoned with salt-free spices, then baked and served with lean protein and steamed green vegetables, that's perfect. However, if a potato is slathered with butter and bacon bits, loaded with salt and paired with a fatty steak, the meal is no longer healthy for your liver.

The next step is understanding the top foods your liver needs and those that it needs to avoid. In this way you'll know what to load up on your plate, and what to pass up. It can be easy to make small adjustments and additives to your daily diet that are delicious and savory, while avoiding some of the common foods that will negatively impact your liver and slow down your progress to healing NAFLD or NASH. Use this list as a guide to jump into recipe books or food-based websites to find meals that will use these ingredients, and show you how to cook recipes or order dishes that you'll look forward to eating every day. We'll start by going over some of the healthiest foods for your liver.

Garlic

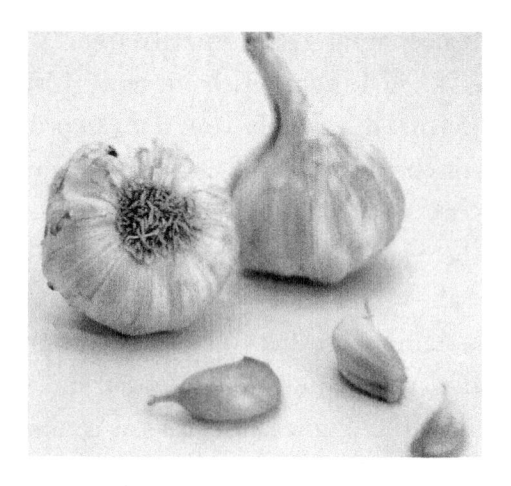

For a small, pungent bulb, this root has a multitude of health benefits. The most important benefit for those with a fatty liver is the components in garlic that promote optimal immune health as well as encourage the liver to cleanse itself. Garlic contains multiple active compounds that can affect your liver health, namely S-allyl cysteine (SAC), S-allylmercaptocysteine (SAMC), diallyl disulfide (DADS), and cinnamoyloctopamines. Don't worry if these names are hard to remember, as generally a garlic supplement or whole garlic will contain all of them! Among the amazing effects of garlic on liver cells are its ability to activate SIRT1, which reduces the production of ROS, reduces the liver's ability to make new fats, and prevents liver cells from killing themselves as a result of damage. SAMC and DADS specifically can also fight liver fibrosis by reducing cellular levels of proteins associated with inflammation, as well as those that activate the inflammatory Kupffer cells that encourage collagen buildup.

Finally, SAMC can activate cellular pathways associated with liver cells' ability to regulate how much fat they carry, and also works to reduce insulin resistance (Perumpail et al., 2018). One study on rats demonstrated that a diet high in garlic could help reduce the harm to the rats' livers from a high-fructose diet. The rats who ate diets with extra garlic showed less oxidative stress, improved fat metabolism in the liver, and less insulin resistance when compared to the control group (Xiao et al., 2013).

Ginger

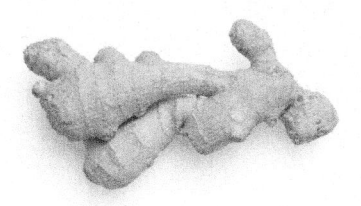

Ginger, a common counterpart to garlic, is almost as popular in world cuisines and included in a number of traditional medicinal practices. Ginger is commonly added to teas, used for flavoring in dishes, and even made into candy throughout different cultures. There is evidence that ginger has strong anti-inflammatory and antioxidant properties that could make it a beneficial part of any liver-healthy supplement routine. For example, ginger boosts the cell's ability to neutralize reactive oxygen radicals, while also reducing cellular levels of a number of signaling proteins associated with inflammation, including the very potent inflammatory signaler TNF-alpha. A study on 44 volunteers with NAFLD demonstrated that the group who took ginger supplements experienced better outcomes than the group who did not, including reduced fat buildup in the liver and reduced insulin resistance (Perumpail et al., 2018).

Lemon

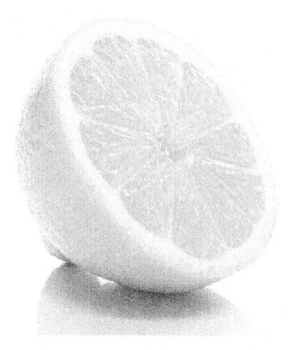

This super sour fruit is known for its high antioxidant agents as well as being high in vitamin C, both of which are excellent for liver health. Under TCM, sour foods are thought to be especially nourishing to the liver. Lemon juice is also a part of Ayurveda, where it is known to improve digestion. The only negative is that they are very acidic and can hurt the stomach in high doses. But lemon is just as good watered down a bit, drizzled on salads, or used in cooking to add a bit of freshness.

Leafy Greens

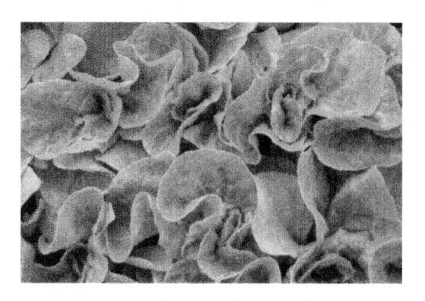

Dark green, leafy vegetables like spinach and kale are packed with fiber, antioxidants, and other compounds that are great for your liver. They also include bioactive compounds called polyphenols that come with a range of health benefits. Raw greens are usually more helpful than cooked greens, so try to eat salads as much as possible!

Green Tea

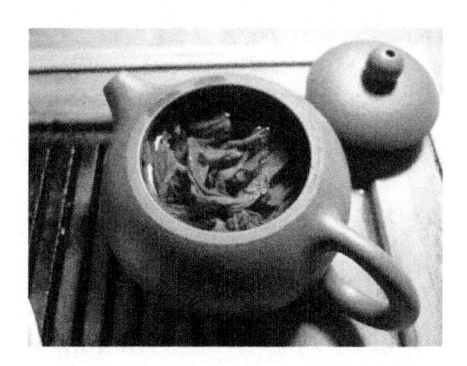

This popular tea contains vitamin C, antioxidants, polyphenols, and other valuable nutrients. It also contains caffeine, which can help control liver enzymes. Green tea is commonly included as part of treatment plans that incorporate TCM.

Carrots and Beets

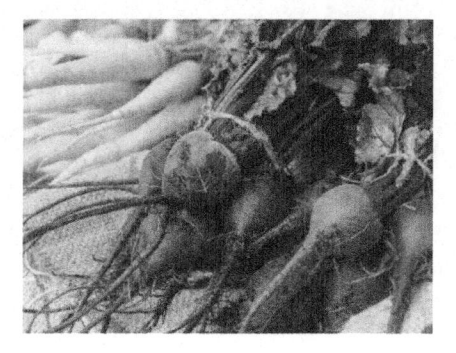

These sweet root vegetables are two of the most nutritious vegetables for your liver. They are packed with anti-inflammatory and antioxidant compounds that can help soothe the effects of NAFLD. You can roast these healthy vegetables, add them to soups, or shred them into salads.

Avocados

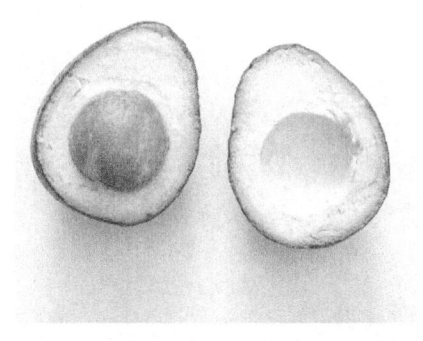

This amazing fruit has so many liver-friendly aspects. Not only are they high in unsaturated fats, which are much better for your liver than saturated fats, they are also packed with fiber which helps to improve digestion.

Nuts and Seeds

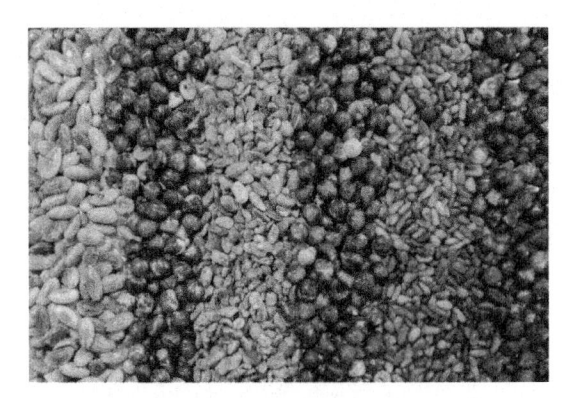

Nuts are packed with unsaturated fats and other nutrients that are important to your liver health. They can also work to fight oxidative stress and reduce inflammation. They're great raw as a snack or added to stir-fries, salads, or healthy baked treats. You may also want to include flax, sunflower, and chia seeds in your diet. These powerful and tasty seeds are packed with omega-3 acids and can also work to lower fat buildup in the liver.

Low-fat Cow's Milk

Individuals with fatty liver disease have to add more calcium intake to their diets. The lower fat kinds, or almond or soy milks, can provide you with vital calcium and vitamin D, both of which your liver needs to function. Those with advanced liver disease often have nutritional depletions which can also put them at a risk for other conditions, such as osteoporosis. These risks can be reduced by getting enough calcium.

Coffee

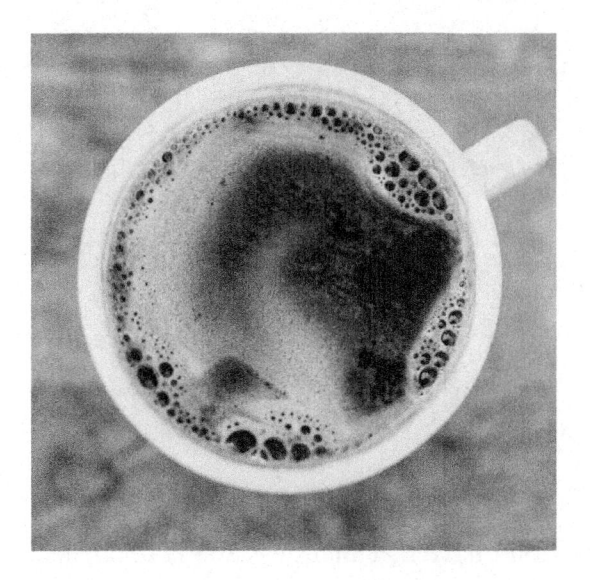

Skip the cream and sugar, and this beverage is a power drink commonly recommended to people coping with NAFLD. Coffee can help reduce your risk of fibrosis and lower blood levels of harmful liver enzymes. If you don't enjoy the bitterness of coffee, you can always find naturally-flavored versions as long as there is no added sugar.

Unsaturated Oils

Some oils actually help to reduce liver enzymes and give the liver much-needed good fats. The oils to reach for include olive, avocado, sesame, sunflower, vegetable, and safflower. These oils are also great if you're trying to lose weight, as they encourage your body to secrete satiety hormones that make you feel satisfied after a meal.

Oatmeal

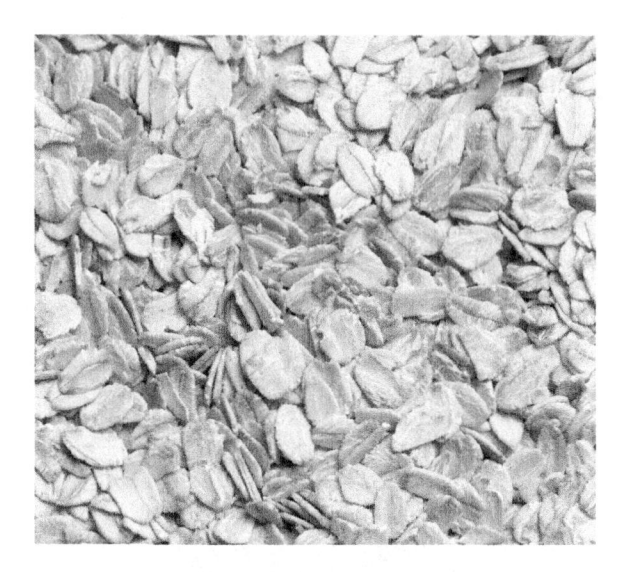

This fiber-rich breakfast favorite helps to reduce the triglyceride fats in the liver, making it one of the more important foods to eat regularly for NAFLD individuals.

Fatty Fish

Those who don't have fish allergies can greatly benefit from the anti-inflammatory properties of these foods, which are packed with omega-3s and other healthy fats. Salmon, trout, sardines, and tuna are all high in omega-3 fatty acids, which help to reduce liver fat, cholesterol, and triglycerides. These fish are also very satisfying to eat, which is also helpful when it comes to losing weight. Finally, omega-3s are essential for your brain health, which is something you want to be conscious of if you're experiencing problems with your liver. Hepatic encephalophy is a neurological syndrome that occurs when a liver can't do its work, so promoting good brain health is a prudent move when your liver isn't working correctly.

Beans and Soy Products

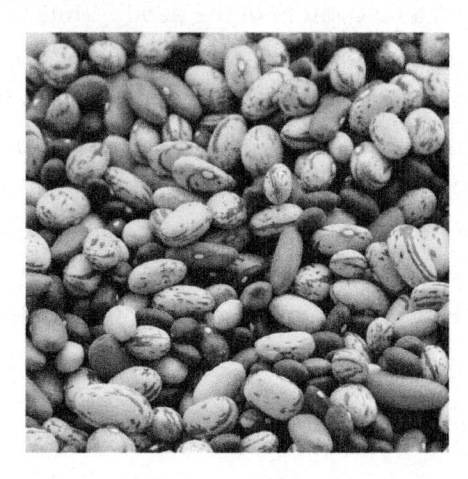

These are the foods to turn to when trying to reduce your meat intake, as many meats are packed with unhealthy saturated fats. Tofu is a great low-fat protein source for people coping with NAFLD.

Your Liver-Healthy Diet: Foods to Avoid

Now that the most healthy options have been covered, the list of the most harmful will be included here. Most of these foods are high in saturated fats, sodium, and/or sugar, which places strain on your liver when it's not working correctly.

Fatty Cuts of Meat

Fatty cuts of meat are usually packed with saturated fats. For example, the marbling in a cut of beef or pork is entirely made of saturated fats, which have been shown to be worse for your liver than unsaturated fats. Remember, fatty liver disease is an indication that there is too much fat building up in your liver cells. Therefore, you want to limit how much fat you're taking in through your diet in general, but due to the uniquely poor health effects associated with saturated fats, you're going to want to avoid them in particular.

Which foods are especially high in saturated fats? In particular, you're going to want to avoid red meat, which includes beef, veal, and pork, as well as dairy and eggs. You should also avoid fattier cuts of chicken and other white meat, like the thighs. Leaving the skin on chicken also sharply increases the saturated fat content of the meal. While many people look at this list and assume they'll have to go completely vegan, you can still enjoy leaner cuts of chicken and other white meats in limited amounts. For example, chicken breast has a much lower fat content than liver thighs, wings, and drumsticks. In order to reduce the fat content of your meal in general, roast your chicken instead of frying it and choose low-fat options for flavoring. For example, rubbing your chicken with spices (consider using some that are listed as healthy for your liver in the next chapter!) is a healthier option than using a sauce packed with fat and sugar.

Furthermore, if your medical provider does recommend you go vegetarian or vegan for your liver health, this isn't the end of the world: There is not a single amino acid found in animals that you cannot find in plants as well, so you won't be malnourished. Furthermore, there is evidence that getting too much of some amino acids can be harmful to your body (Garlick, 2004), and that the lower amounts found in plant foods are actually helpful to you. If you decide to strongly reduce the amount of meat in your diet or forgo it completely, be sure to eat a variety of beans, lentils, nuts, and seeds to make sure you get all the protein you need for your health.

Cured and Processed Meats

Just like the types of meat we described above, cured and processed meats are packed with saturated fats and sodium. In fact, salt is an integral part of the process of creating these addictive but unhealthy foods! While salt is the reason that bacon, sausages, prosciutto, salami, pepperoni, and processed sandwich meats taste great, it's also very harmful for your liver, especially if you're dealing with a case of NAFLD. In fact, a 2016 study published by Choi et al. showed that people who eat diets high in sodium increase their risk for NAFLD overall. This was done by analyzing the data from liver ultrasonography of over 100,000 volunteers, and comparing this data to the volunteers' diets. When the results were adjusted for body weight, the correlation was less stark, but still significant. It's possible that a diet high in sodium is even more dangerous to people carrying a few extra pounds, but if you have NAFLD, you should avoid these foods as much as possible regardless of your weight.

Junk Food

Junk food and processed snacks such as chips, cookies, candy, and sodas are not good for your health even when you don't have a liver condition, and if you're suffering from NAFLD, these should be cut out of your diet as much as possible. Many of these foods are packed with sugars, including fructose, which is one of the worst things you can consume for your liver health. In fact, a diet high in fructose is one of the most prominent risk factors for NAFLD and NASH, as it promotes fat synthesis in the liver. High-fructose corn syrup is a common sweetener in sodas and other kinds of junk food, but any kind of fructose is harmful for your liver.

Furthermore, fructose isn't the only kind of sugar that can harm your liver: Any kind of refined sugar found in packaged treats increases your risk of obesity, insulin resistance, and type II diabetes, all of which increase your risk for NAFLD and make it harder to recover. Many packaged snacks are often high in saturated fats, which are used in the preparation of pastries, cookies, and similar products. Saturated fats are worse for your liver than unsaturated fats, so this presents another reason why these kinds of treats should be avoided if at all possible.

Deep-Fried Foods

While canola oil, the most common oil used for deep frying, is very low in saturated fats and contains many unsaturated fats, deep-fried foods are generally not recommended for people who are dealing with NAFLD. First of all, while unsaturated fats are not as bad for your liver as saturated fats, you should still limit the amount of fat in your diet overall. Furthermore, a lot of deep-fried foods found at places such as McDonald's, KFC, and similar fast-food brands are extremely high in sodium, which can worsen NAFLD outcomes regardless of your weight. Finally, eating fast-foods or other deep-fried foods is linked to obesity, which is one of the main risk factors for NAFLD. If you really miss eating fried foods, why not look for a baked or roasted low-sodium alternative to your favorite recipe?

Cooking Oils and Fats

Common fats used for cooking include coconut oil, butter, margarine, hydrogenated vegetable oil, and lard. These foods, while extremely useful in cooking and as condiments, are unfortunately made of saturated fats. Saturated fats have been shown to be worse for your liver health than unsaturated fats, so you don't want to have too much of these in your diet when you're trying to reverse NAFLD.

While you should opt for low-fat meals when dealing with fatty liver disease, this requirement is not as strict when it comes to olive oil and other oils made of unsaturated fats. In fact, unsaturated fats can be generally good for your health: this is why our Fatty Liver Diet Plan recommends you continue to eat avocados! Therefore, opt for olive oil or another unsaturated oil when you need to use an oil for cooking, for salad dressings, or as a condiment.

Refined Carbohydrates

Refined carbohydrates in this context refer to the very simple carbs found in white bread and white pasta. While whole-grain bread contains more complex carbs and fiber—meaning that the sugar from these foods is released into the bloodstream more gradually—the carbs in white bread and pasta are digested very quickly, leading to a rush of sugar into the bloodstream shortly after consumption. Eating too many simple carbs over time can lead to insulin resistance, one of the warning signs for type II diabetes, a risk factor for NAFLD. Since simple carbs are processed very quickly by the body, they are not a great option for satisfying your hunger, and you can eat way more calories than you mean to if your meal is mostly made of them. This can lead to overeating, especially if you feel hungry again a short time later. Overeating can lead to excess weight gain, another major risk factor for NAFLD. If you must eat grains, opt for whole-grain varieties as much as possible.

Full-fat Dairy

This includes full-fat cream, milk, butter, and cheese. These foods are extremely high in fats, leading to problems if your liver isn't producing bile to emulsify them correctly. Furthermore, most of the fats in these groups consist of saturated fats, which should be removed from your diet as much as possible when you're struggling with NAFLD. A suitable alternative to dairy products in your liver-healthy diet could be nut milks such as almond milk instead of cow's milk, olive oil for cooking instead of butter, and soy-based vegan cheeses (look for a low-sugar variety!).

The Fatty Liver Diet Program

Now that you know some of the specific foods to include or avoid, let's put it together into an easy, everyday plan. How can you use what you've learned to make a healthy shopping list and meal plan for the week?

First, let's start with what you're buying at the grocery store. Make yourself a list of the ingredients you need to keep stocked in your pantry, such as the ones mentioned above, to avoid impulse buying foods that could further damage your fatty liver. Make sure to plan for cravings and snacks—it's better to know what you can snack on ahead of time instead of rushing to the corner store when you want junk food. Pick low-sugar fruits and healthy vegetables high in fiber. While we mentioned the need to avoid fructose on the fatty liver diet, new research shows that fruits lower in sugar can have a positive effect on fatty liver because of the amount of fiber and antioxidants contained in them (Gyimah, 2021). Just remember to choose fruits such as apples, raspberries, and cantaloupe rather than mangoes, watermelon, and bananas. Other great snacks to add in are roasted nuts, nut butters, or hummus as they contain healthy fats and pair great with apples and carrots. If you know you like to eat crunchy treats, choose at-home air-popped popcorn (with a small amount of olive oil if desired) and kale or kelp chips—these should be eaten only once in a while, but they are a better option than greasy potato chips or flavored popcorn. You will also want to get in the habit of checking product labels to avoid hidden additives that increase sugar and trans fat and would be harmful on the fatty liver diet.

If you find it hard to come up with ideas of what to create each week to keep meals interesting and healthy, read on for some simple suggestions that many with fatty liver disease have found helpful.

The best way to start your morning hydration on the fatty liver diet is by drinking a large glass of lemon water. This will give your digestive system a great boost and as we mentioned earlier, lemon is packed full of liver-nourishing properties. Follow this up with oatmeal, one of the best breakfast foods for your fatty liver—it contains protein and extra fiber, and it helps your liver to metabolize unhealthy fats. Unfortunately, you might have bad memories of eating oatmeal or porridge, or think that it is boring and tasteless, but these next suggestions will help you enjoy having it for breakfast! A favorite boost for your liver is to add nuts and seeds to your oatmeal, or mix in cooked quinoa in a 50/50 ratio. While avoiding sweeteners such as brown sugar or maple syrup, use sweeteners such as fresh diced apple or stevia. Studies have found that stevia can even have a protective benefit for those with fatty liver disease, helping metabolize glucose and lipids (Kakleas et. al., 2020). Still, breakfast isn't complete without a hot beverage, so add in a mug of green tea or coffee to your morning routine, skipping the cream for a low-fat milk or dairy substitute; now you're on track for a successful dietary day!

When it comes to lunches, you might need to think outside the box for some fresh solutions. If you usually like to eat sandwiches, it's important to pick lean meats including turkey, or fish such as salmon and tuna. Your liver will thank you even more if you substitute your bread for lettuce, and add in avocado, carrots, or your other favorite vegetables. If you have time to do extra meal preparation during the week, consider taking the time to make something different, such as a roasted beet salad. By using canned beets (without additives), you can prepare this dish more quickly; you can use the beets as is or roast them for extra flavor. Play with different ingredients until you find what you like best, but a classic combination is to add cooked quinoa, kimchi or pickles, tofu, and a roasted garlic and balsamic vinaigrette dressing. This salad is a great way to get the benefits of probiotics, lean protein, and antioxidants in your fatty liver diet.

When it comes to dinner, there are many healthy options for you, including soups and stews. Consider making a meatless yellow pea soup, bean chili with chicken breast, or lentil and spinach soup to get your protein and vitamin needs. If your usual dinner consists of a traditional meat and potato dish, learn to choose lean proteins such as turkey and chicken breast, fish, and tofu. It's important to keep an eye on correct portion sizes and pay attention to what you choose to make for your side dishes. As was mentioned earlier, this may mean that while you can keep your favorites, you may need to change your cooking method. For example, avoid deep-frying or cooking in fats, and instead, opt for boiling, steaming, or braising in low-sodium broth. Again, make sure to keep your portion sizes in line with your doctor's recommended calorie intake. This often means increasing the percentage of vegetables on your plate, and decreasing starchy, sugary side dishes. Remember to have fun with your meals and look for a variety of cuisines to keep it interesting—you can try out sushi bowls, stir-fries, and curries to get loads of vegetables and lean proteins.

Now the tough part: snacks and desserts. While these are tempting to most of us, do your best to stop or limit your intake of unhealthy snacks by changing your choices. Pick low-fat, low-sugar options when possible, although if you are using sugar substitutes, remember to avoid artificial sweeteners and use stevia instead. Make sure to keep vegetables, low-sugar fruits, and nuts on hand for quick and healthy alternative snacks.

There you have it: these are the basic starting points for your new meal plan, and a healthy, tasty way to begin healing your fatty liver!

PART V

Cleanses and Detox for Fatty Liver

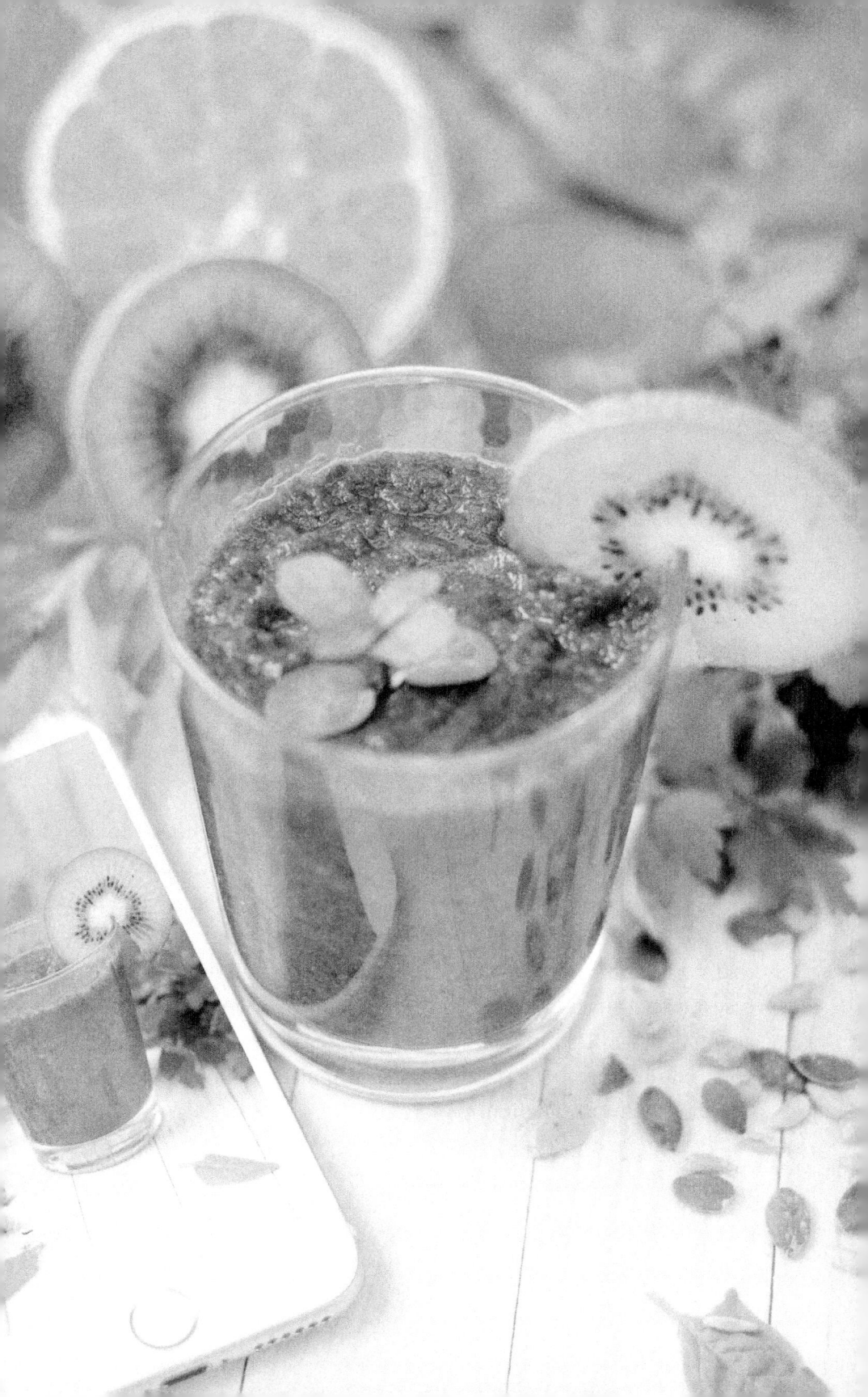

Chapter 7

Natural Remedies for Fatty Liver Disease

As described in previous chapters, people choose to opt for natural remedies for fatty liver disease and other conditions for a diverse range of reasons. Similarly, the people who choose to incorporate natural remedies into their treatment plans are just as diverse, and come from all walks of life. Depending on your particular case of fatty liver disease, your doctor may or may not recommend aggressive medical intervention; even if they do prescribe medication for your condition, you can also look into using natural treatments in conjunction to medication!

Remember, the holistic philosophy of medicine is about treating the whole person: It's not just about using a treatment that targets your liver, but about taking into account the fact that your body is made of inextricably interconnected systems, which all need to be considered. Holistic medicine also allows for you to use both natural or mainstream medications, allowing you the broadest range of options and the most comprehensive treatment possible. Therefore, please follow your doctor's instructions regarding which mainstream medical treatments to take, especially if your liver disease is particularly advanced or severe! A holistic doctor, as well as many mainstream doctors, will be willing to work with you to incorporate both natural and mainstream interventions into your treatment.

Before starting any kind of treatment for an illness, it's important to talk to the medical professionals on your care team. This includes your primary physician as well as any other professionals such as naturopaths or nutritionists who are involved in the care of your liver, and who may be able to point you in the right direction regarding which treatments would be the most beneficial.

Liver Cleanses

To explain how this kind of natural treatment for fatty liver disease works, we need to return to the idea of your liver as the filter for the rest of your body. The purpose of a cleanse or detox is to boost the liver's ability to clear out the toxins and other harmful substances that have built up inside it. The idea is that once your liver has been cleansed, it'll be more free to do its job once you move back into eating normally. This is done by consuming only foods that boost the liver's function, usually while forgoing other foods and fasting in between doses. The process usually takes place over a period of a few days.

So what's the evidence that this can help? While modern medicine provides some evidence for the use of cleanses in that it agrees that some ingredients of liver cleanses and detoxes can be helpful to your liver health (see more on this below), the practice is also drawn from Ayurveda and TCM principles. For example, in Ayurveda, the liver is thought to be the part of the body that holds negative emotions as well as physical toxins, and cleansing the liver is thought to help clear these out to improve your health. In TCM, the liver is thought to help regulate the vital energy known as *qi*, and blood that is filtered by the liver is thought to carry *qi* around the body, so detoxing the liver is thought to be beneficial for the body as a whole.

Liver cleanses can be a controversial topic with research to determine their effectiveness still underway. However, most scientists agree that many common ingredients in liver cleanses can be good for your liver, and potentially activate biochemical pathways or perform other functions that can help fight NAFLD. Furthermore, many liver cleanses involve fasting between the servings of juice, and fasting can be a great way to help yourself lose weight when done in a healthy manner. So long as you clear your liver cleanse with your physician or other medical professional, there's no reason you shouldn't try it!

It's important to talk to your medical team before performing a liver cleanse, and take their advice. Liver cleanses are not appropriate for everyone, and can be dangerous for some individuals. Below, we've included a list of people who should not perform a liver cleanse, while acknowledging that this list is not exhaustive and that everyone should listen to the advice of a medical professional regarding whether or not a liver cleanse is appropriate for them:

- people who are malnourished or underweight
- people who are diabetic or otherwise struggle to regulate blood sugar
- people who are pregnant, postpartum, or breastfeeding
- people in extremely hot or cold climates
- people undergoing a lot of emotional stress
- people who are prone to fainting when hungry
- people dealing with infections or illnesses
- people on a special diet for any medical issue

Remember also that a cleanse or detox won't be able to fix NAFLD or another liver disease all by itself. It's still extremely important to lose weight, change your diet, get some exercise, and otherwise make the lifestyle changes suggested by your medical team. However, a cleanse or detox can be a valued part of your liver health plan, when combined with other interventions to cover your bases as broadly as possible.

Below, we've included a list of ingredients that you may want to include in your liver cleanse or detox, with notes on the evidence for their efficacy.

Apple Cider Vinegar

Apple cider vinegar is one of the hottest topics in health and lifestyle circles these days, and it's not hard to see why. Apple cider vinegar has a number of scientifically supported health benefits, including helping with lowering blood sugar and blood cholesterol. Apple cider vinegar has also been shown by a recent study to help prevent liver damage in rats who were fed with a diet high in fats (Bouazza et al., 2015). While more research is needed on humans to confirm its effectiveness, apple cider vinegar is commonly included in liver detox recipes, or can be drunk on its own out of a shot glass!

Beetroot

Beetroots are one of the sweetest-tasting vegetables, and also carry a number of health benefits for your liver under the principles of both Western and traditional medicines, including Ayurveda. Beetroot has anti-inflammatory properties that could help to combat chronic hepatitis, as well as antioxidant properties that could help combat oxidative stress in the liver. One certified Ayurveda practitioner suggests that eating beetroot could help boost the natural detoxification enzymes in your liver (Sahoo, 2021). All of these benefits are also supported by modern science, and several trials have been done in recent years to confirm their efficacy. For one example, a 2015 review chronicled years of studies demonstrating that beetroot has both anti-inflammatory and antioxidant properties (Clifford et al., 2015).

Carrot

While the common notion that carrots are good for your eyes is actually a myth, these popular veggies are actually great for your liver, and taste particularly great if you enjoy savory juices! One of the active compounds in carrots is retinoic acid, a nutrient that works to regulate inflammation. One study conducted in 2012 suggests that carrots can help reduce hepatitis by reducing inflammatory-signaling proteins in immune cells in the liver (Nagy, 2012). The benefits don't stop there: Another study showed that, while carrots did not seem to lower fat levels in the liver, they could reduce some blood markers of liver damage (Mahesh et al., 2016).

Apple

Who doesn't love apple juice? Along with being sweet and satisfying, apples and apple juice can be great additions to a liver cleanse. Apple juice has been shown by scientific studies to be packed with polyphenols, which are natural biological compounds with a range of health benefits. In the case of liver health, one study showed that a diet high in apple juice polyphenols reduced markers of liver damage in blood work done on rats (Krajka-Kuźniak et al., 2015).

There's only one catch: The clear apple juice you buy at the store isn't the best for this. Cloudy apple juice, which still contains pulp that store brands usually remove, has four times as many polyphenols as clear apple juice (Society of Chemical Industry, 2007). To get the most out of the apple juice in your liver cleanse, buy a few of your favorite breed of apple and juice them at home!

Dandelion Root

Dandelion root has been used in a number of traditional medicine practices in the past to handle liver issues like hepatitis and jaundice, and its benefits for the liver are well known under Western medicine as well. One study from 2017 suggested that dandelion root could protect your liver from damage as a result of acetaminophen and other toxic compounds (Cai et al., 2017). It can also reduce inflammation, though this is a milder effect than that of some of the other ingredients on this list (Wong, 2021). Dandelion root is best known in TCM as a diuretic, and encourages your body to clear toxins and other unwanted substances through urination. This herb is also believed to be nourishing to the liver under the principles of TCM. You can make a tea out of dandelion root, let it cool, and then mix it into your liver cleansing juice.

Turmeric

Through its active component curcumin, turmeric is one of the healthiest spices on the market, and has been lauded by both natural and Western medical practitioners for its health benefits. Turmeric supplements are all the rage as of late (see the section on supplementation below), and for good reason.

Under TCM, turmeric is a go-to substance for decongesting and detoxing the liver. Western medicine also supports its effects: Turmeric has strong anti-inflammatory properties, and helps to reduce fat buildup in the liver. More information on turmeric's liver benefits can be found in the following chapter.

Finally, adding turmeric to your liver cleanse juice can add a savory zing to the flavor, as well as turn it a very appealing bright yellow color. While this part doesn't help your liver, it can definitely make a liver cleanse juice more fun to drink!

Magnolia Berry

Magnolia berry has anti-inflammatory properties, which makes it a helpful addition to your liver cleanse routine if you're worried about chronic hepatitis. It is also rich in antioxidants, allowing you to prevent damage to your liver through reactive oxygen species produced as a side product of metabolism. Finally, magnolia berry may be able to lessen the liver-toxic effects of acetaminophen, making it a great choice if you've only recently removed Tylenol or generic brands from your medicine cabinet.

Finally, remember to drink plenty of water, exercise, and take care of your emotional health while undergoing a liver cleanse. Most alternative and holistic medical practices acknowledge the importance of the emotional and spiritual parts of human existence when treating physical ailments. It can be helpful to have a good cry when you're feeling stressed or sad, talk to loved ones, and perform yoga or another relaxing activity to reduce stress. Going for a brisk walk or spending time in nature can also be good for your mental and physical health when dealing with a liver issue, and be especially helpful with regards to staying positive.

Herbal and Other Supplements

While we've already touched on the importance of certain foods in your liver-friendly diet, as well as how including certain foods in your diet can help to combat or reverse NAFLD, there's also emerging evidence that taking herbal supplements can help to treat this scary condition as well. While there are no currently prescribed diagnostics to cure NAFLD, recent studies suggest that certain herbal therapies can work to reverse the disease, or at least to slow its progression. The information in this section comes from four scientific reviews on the effectiveness of herbal supplements to treat NAFLD. A review is a peer-reviewed scientific paper, published in an established journal, that examines the current evidence around a certain topic and synthesizes this information into a conclusion. The reviews we will be citing selected which herbs to investigate based on which have been used in alternative medical practices, including TCM and Ayurvedic medicine, but each study cited in the review included rigorous scientific experimentation to investigate the benefits of each product.

Before including herbal supplements in your fatty liver disease treatment plan, it's important to speak to your medical provider. Not every supplement is appropriate for every person, and taking the wrong supplement can do much more harm to your liver than good.

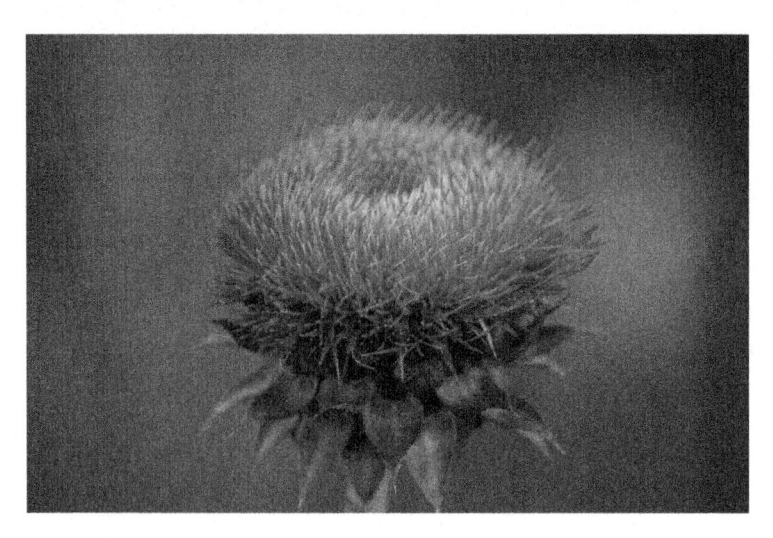

Milk Thistle

Milk thistle is a wild-growing plant that is commonly used in supplements marketed to people with liver problems. This is one of the most effective supplement components on the market today, and should be at the top of most people's lists when it comes to formulating a liver-healthy supplement routine. Furthermore, due to the incredible amount of evidence in mouse trials for milk thistle's effects on fatty liver, numerous human trials have been initiated and are ongoing, with promising early results.

The active ingredient in milk thistle extract is a compound called silymarin, which is responsible for the plants ability to combat NAFLD. There are three main components to silymarin's action on the liver: its antioxidant properties, its ability to reduce fat accumulation, and its ability to reduce inflammation.

Antioxidants have been lauded for their health benefits in recent years, though research is still ongoing and the subject of some controversy. Normal cell metabolism produces reactive oxygen species (ROS), which carry an extra electron and can damage cells and DNA. Your body contains natural mechanisms to combat ROS buildup, but many natural health practitioners also recommend that patients take antioxidants or incorporate antioxidant foods into their diets. Antioxidants have the ability to neutralize ROS, protecting your cells. Silymarin is well established as an antioxidant, as it activates biochemical pathways that protect the cell by boosting the function of natural antioxidant enzymes (Xiao et al., 2013).

Silymarin can also help fight fat buildup in the liver by restoring the IRS-1/PI3K/Akt pathway, which also fights insulin resistance, a symptom of type II diabetes and also a risk factor for NAFLD. It also reduces the liver's ability to synthesize new fats by activating another chemical pathway. The anti-inflammatory effects of milk thistle are just as well-known, and the plant activates a number of biochemical processes that can soothe chronic inflammation. Specifically, it works to inhibit the action of Nf-kB, an intracellular signaling molecule that regulates the inflammatory reaction (Perumpail et al., 2018).

Ginkgo Biloba

Ginkgo biloba is a common ingredient in traditional Chinese medicines, and in recent years a significant amount of scientific research has been dedicated to exploring its properties. Commonly lauded for its antioxidant properties, the leaves of this fascinating plant may also be able to prevent the buildup of fats in the liver.

Ginkgo biloba has been shown to boost the activity of an intracellular compound called CPT-1A, which improves liver cells' ability to regulate the amount of fat building up in the organ. Furthermore, like silymarin, ginkgo biloba has antioxidant properties in that it prevents the production of ROS while also boosting the cell's natural antioxidant enzymes (Perumpail et al., 2018). While human trials are still ongoing, early experiments on mice suggest that ginkgo biloba is a great addition to your toolbox when developing a liver-healthy supplement regimen.

Resveratrol

Resveratrol is a polyphenol, or a type of chemically active compound found in plants. Many polyphenols are good for you, but resveratrol is the most famous of them, and has been repeatedly cited for its ability to fight inflammation and improve your cardiac health. Since so much of liver disease is centered around inflammation, there's no wonder that people have started to investigate whether resveratrol can be helpful to your liver as well.

Resveratrol has been extensively tested for its ability to improve your liver health, mostly in mouse models, though research on humans is ongoing and showing promising results. The authors of one extensive review compare resveratrol to milk thistle, in that it has potent anti-inflammatory and antioxidant effects. Resveratrol is well-known to activate the AMK/SIRT1 pathway which has a vast range of benefits including reducing inflammation, improving your liver's ability to metabolize fat, and inducing autophagy, a renewing process that allows cells to eat and digest toxins and other unwanted compounds. Resveratrol has also been shown to reduce markers of cellular stress, preventing cells from killing themselves through a process known as apoptosis (Perumpail et al., 2018). Another review found that resveratrol prevents the activation of genes involved in the liver's ability to synthesize fats (Xiao et al., 2013).

Resveratrol is naturally found in red wine, grapes, and olive oil, and is one of the main reasons that all of these foods are considered good for your heart. However, drinking alcohol is a terrible idea when you have fatty liver disease, and you should not take up red wine as a way to include resveratrol in your diet. Instead, opt for nonalcoholic foods that contain the compound, or take it as an extraneous supplement.

Turmeric

We've already mentioned this iconic yellow spice in this book, but we felt it was worth bringing up here! The active compound in turmeric is curcumin, and this is the compound that you'll actually be taking if you choose to include turmeric supplements in your diet plan.

Curcumin has a potent ability to reduce oxidative stress by neutralizing ROS before they can do much damage. Furthermore, this fascinating compound can help regulate how much fat is stored in the liver by activating biochemical pathways associated with the liver's ability to remove excess fats. Finally, curcumin is able to help regulate intracellular levels of signaling proteins involved in the inflammatory process, which means that taking this supplement can also help you reduce liver inflammation (Perumpail et al., 2018).

The main thing to remember when you're taking a turmeric supplement is that you need to take black pepper as well to ensure that your body can absorb curcumin properly. This is essential if you want to get your money's worth. If you're taking an extraneous turmeric supplement, be sure to choose one that also contains black pepper extract. If you choose instead to simply add more turmeric to your food (a low-fat curry with a plant protein like lentils is a great liver-healthy meal, and a great way to eat more turmeric!), be sure to give your plate a good few cracks of black pepper as well!

Ursolic and Carnosic Acid

These two acids are chemically active compounds found in a range of household herbs that are commonly used as flavorings for meat and other dishes. These herbs include basil, sage, peppermint, lavender, oregano, and rosemary. While they are often listed together, because common herb combinations result in both of them being included in the same recipes and because some herbs contain them both, these compounds can actually improve your liver health in completely different ways. Ursolic acid reduces intracellular stress signals, which lowers inflammation and prevents the cell from killing itself through apoptosis. It also improves liver cells' ability to regulate the amount of fat they carry by activating AMPK and other relevant biochemical pathways. On the other hand, carnosic acid reduces intracellular levels of proteins associated with inflammation, as well as preventing apoptosis by reducing levels of proteins associated with this process. Carsonic acid also has antioxidant effects, preventing the buildup of ROS in the cell (Perumpail et al., 2018).

Goji Berry

Goji berries have been used in Chinese medicine to treat liver disease, helping manage the health of the liver and prevent further progression of NAFLD. Known as a superfood, they are made up of chemical compounds called phytochemicals that contain polysaccharides, beta-carotene, and zeaxanthin. These three compounds work together to boost the body's immune system and improve antioxidant activity as a whole (Barhum, 2018). It can be simple to bring them into your diet as they're so versatile and simple to get access to. Including goji berries in your smoothies, salads, whole grains, and snacks will make enjoying the benefits of this fruit easy and simple.

Castor Oil

The website associated with one naturopathic practice mentions the use of castor oil packs (Morstein, 2010), which means applying castor oil externally (sometimes with heat) to help decongest and cleanse the liver. Using a castor oil pack can help improve circulation while also helping it eliminate toxins from your body. There are a couple different schools of thought around how to make castor oil packs, but one instruction set recommends cutting wool or cotton flannel into three 12 in. by 14 in. pieces, stacking them together, and saturating them in castor oil. It's important to keep adding castor oil until the flannel stops absorbing it, which means you may end up using way more oil than you anticipated. Once the flannel is completely soaked, you can heat it up (if desired) by wrapping it in plastic, like a garbage bag, and putting it on top of a heating pad for 15 minutes.

This is the safest way to heat up your castor oil pack without making it hot enough to burn you–never use a microwave for this! Once the pack is warm, place it on your abdomen on top of the liver with the heating pad on top of the pack to keep it warm. Since the pack should be dripping with oil, you may want to put some towels or plastic sheeting underneath you on your bed or couch to prevent a mess. You can keep this on for 60-90 minutes, which can be a great time to meditate if meditation is also part of your NAFLD treatment plan.

Part VI

Seven Rules to Follow for a Healthy Liver

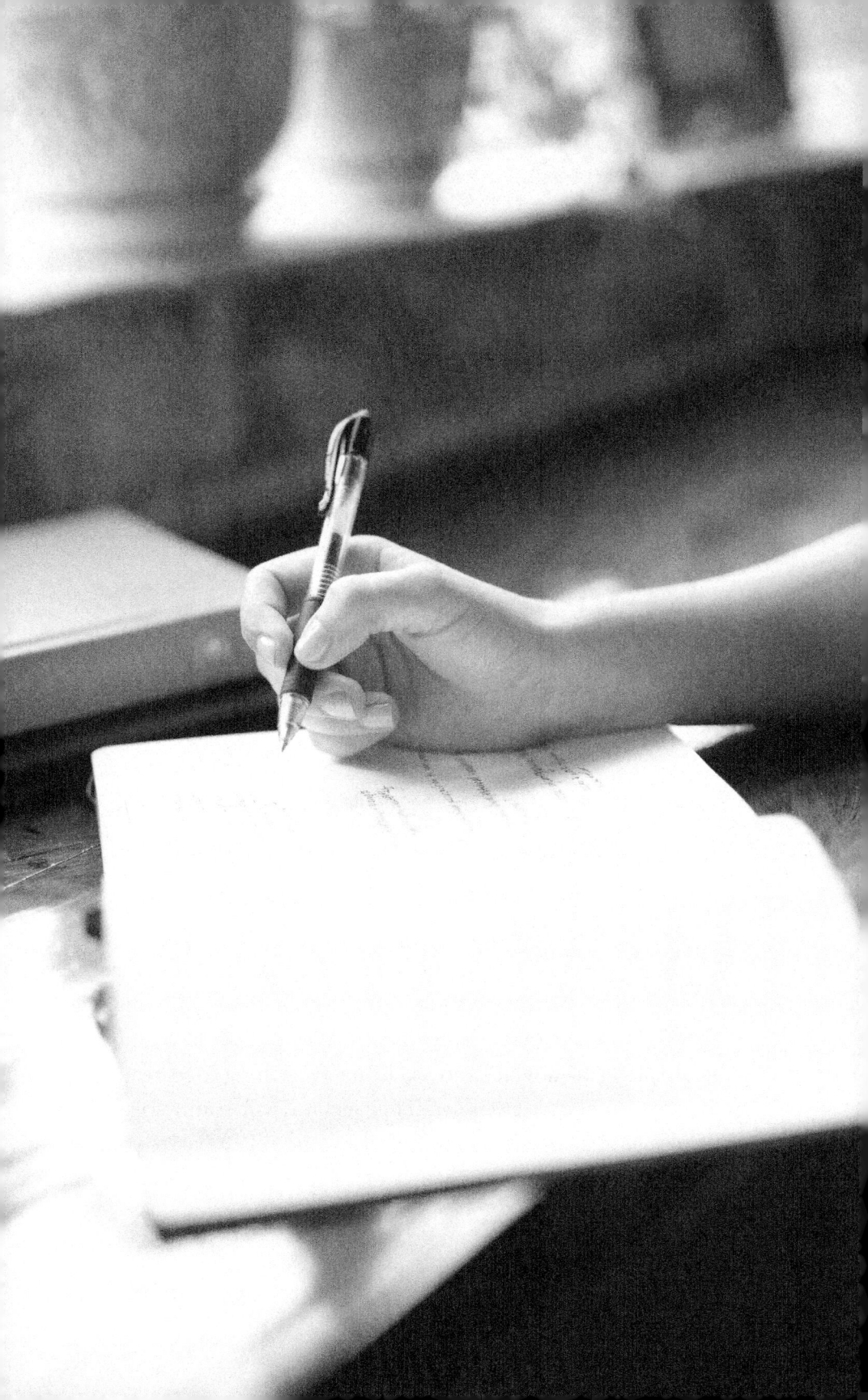

Chapter 8

Seven Steps to Prevent and Reverse Fatty Liver Disease

While NAFLD is a growing epidemic, resulting from an increase in obesity and insulin that creates higher levels of fat in the liver, there are seven steps you can follow to reverse fatty liver disease. We've covered so much in this book already, and now it's time to bring everything together with action steps you can start right now. This section will summarize all of the principles in this book in seven steps, so you can familiarize yourself with each concept. It will also help you get started on the right foot, should you choose to dive in even deeper with your own research outside of this book. Additionally, these seven steps will also help you when you're talking to your doctor, explaining your new lifestyle to your family and friends, and knowing where to get started when setting goals for yourself.

You may think of these steps as near-magic solutions, a list of things to follow that will support your ambitions of healing your liver, and you'd be right. While they cannot be categorized as a true magic bullet solution, following these steps will give you the information, strategy, and support you need to be successful. If, for whatever reason, you've skimmed the earlier sections of this book or perhaps you're a reader that likes to skip to the end first, then this chapter will contain everything you need to go in the correct direction. Following these steps can help prevent and reverse fatty liver disease, empowering you with the information you need to change your lifestyle and enjoy the benefits of having a balanced, healthy liver.

Seven Steps to Reverse NAFLD

These seven magic rules are general guidelines you'll want to follow in various areas of your life. Some reference working with your doctor, others focus on lifestyle changes, while the rest are resources you can invest in to help turn things around. Knowing these steps will help you have an overall understanding of where you need to make changes, ask questions, and learn about more in detail. With knowledge, comes power; having a comprehensive database of information about your liver will help you prevent and reverse NAFLD.

Learn About Your Liver

The liver is a complicated organ, which performs over 500 functions throughout the body. It includes a number of important components, including four lobes, the bile duct, arteries, veins, capillaries, membranes, and several different types of cells including hepatocytes and Kupffer cells. The human body couldn't survive if the liver stopped functioning for even a single day, which is why it's so important that you reverse the side effects of fatty liver disease. While a healthy liver is made up of 10% fat, going over this amount is when the body is at risk to develop type II diabetes and insulin resistance. Your liver stocks up on necessary vitamins and nutrients, like iron, to use later when the body needs it. Perhaps most importantly, the liver is responsible for detoxing anything we ingest that is harmful to our body. Things like alcohol and drugs would not be processed or broken down within the liver; this means the body would treat these things the same way it treats poison or a virus, by attacking it and removing it from the body in forceful, unideal ways.

There are a number of risk factors for fatty liver disease, such as alcohol use, obesity, exposure to toxins, and diabetes. When you are consuming high levels of foods that the liver struggles to digest, it will begin to work less efficiently and be overwhelmed with the workload you're asking it to undertake. Think of fatty liver disease as your liver burning itself out, being unable to perform at its highest function and, even though it needs a break, this is being denied to the liver. Be specific and careful about what you put in your body, and think about the effect it's having on your internal organs, namely the liver. Did you know that it isn't just foods that can negatively impact your liver? There are a range of common products such as acetaminophen (also known as Tylenol), amoxicillin, and any non-steroidal anti-inflammatory drug such as ibuprofen or Naproxen that can harm your liver, but many people don't realize this. You'll want to be careful how much medication you are taking on a daily basis and keep your doctor in the loop when it comes to being honest about what you're taking, how much, and how often. Learning how the liver works and what happens when any of its essential functions are impaired is one of the most important things you can do for yourself when it comes to avoiding, reversing, and managing NAFLD and NASH.

Advocate for Yourself

Once you have the knowledge you need, you can be more confident when talking to your doctor and the rest of your medical team about which treatments would be right for you. There are a lot of options and roads you can take to build the perfect reversal strategy that will work for you. Don't be afraid to speak up and ask questions; if you find that being in the doctor's office is overwhelming or you forget what the doctor says, bring an advocate with you to take notes or ask the doctor if you can record the visit to play it back later. Sometimes being told a large amount of information, with detailed directions all at once can be too much for our mind to fully absorb and remember in its entirety. It's perfectly normal to ask for someone to accompany you or to record the visit to your doctor with the purpose of making sure that you have access to everything the doctor has told you.

Being confident and asking the questions you need to ask allows you to take the reins of your treatment and get the best benefit possible out of every visit to the doctor's office. Don't keep any information back from the doctor when it comes to your lifestyle, hobbies, the food you've been eating, any medication you are on, and what your go-to active or sedentary habits are. Your healthcare team is there to help you evaluate what you've been doing and help build a bridge to what a better lifestyle could be for you. Honesty will help them understand where you are coming from and empower them to give you good advice for how to start making any necessary changes. If at any time you feel overwhelmed with your doctor's instructions, tell them! They are there to listen and direct, as well as to run tests and give a prognosis. After hearing their recommended strategy for positive change, evaluate what treatment sounds like the right fit for you. If you'd like to explore complementary or alternative treatments, tell the doctor and work together to create a strategy that works for you.

Start Losing Weight

Weight loss is part of most NAFLD and NASH treatment plans, as excess fat buildup in the liver lies at the core of the disease. Going over that 10% is detrimental to your liver, which is why something as simple as weight loss can help turn things around. It's not just a good idea for your liver to lose weight and live in a healthy weight range, it is a necessary change that has to happen for your overall quality of life. A great way to get going with your weight-loss plan is to start walking every day for 20-30 minutes. Something as simple as starting, ending, or spending the middle of your day walking will get the weight-loss ball rolling in the right direction and reinforce the habit of exercising or moving every day.

From there, you can start to incorporate different forms of exercise to build strength and challenge your stamina in various muscle groups. You can also adjust your calorie intake, reducing your daily count by 500 calories to promote weight loss. Keep in mind that weight loss comes more from building muscle and regular movement when it is complemented by lean protein, fiber, and healthy vegetables. Restricting your diet or feeling like you're starving yourself is not the goal. In fact, you may find that in changing your staple foods to healthier, nutritious options, you'll be eating more, and feeling more full or satiated while losing weight. Losing weight can help improve your metabolism, lower the fat buildup in your liver, and enable you to make further lifestyle changes such as taking up regular, vigorous exercise. With more stamina, strength, and consistent activity, it will be easier to lose and maintain the right weight range for your body. Weight loss can also help manage conditions like diabetes that can worsen NAFLD. For these reasons, it's important to chat with your medical team about the healthiest way to lose weight and create new, positive habits that will become healthy lifelong behaviors.

Change Your Diet

Along with being an important part of weight loss, there are other reasons why your diet is essential to managing your NAFLD. There are a number of food groups that are essential to include, such as unsaturated fats through fatty fish and plant-based oils; fiber; and anti-inflammatory nutrients and vitamins, including calcium. By following a Mediterranean-style diet, you can make it simple to include most, if not all, of the necessary foods that will help heal and support your liver. Use recipe books, food-focused websites, or your favorite cooking shows to get ideas and follow recipes that sound delicious to you. If cooking isn't something you enjoy or have a lot of time for, you can get creative with the kind of meals you put together, like soups, stews, or salads, that can all be created in large quantities at once and stay fresh for several days. You can also purchase frozen food and use tools like your oven to cook lean meats, allowing you to set a temperature and timer and then walk away until it is finished.

Here's a simple, complete list of the top things you'll want to change in your diet:

- Eliminate all high-fructose corn syrup.
- Remove processed white flour from your diet.
- Stop eating or notably cut down starch.
- Add in healthy fats like olive oil, avocados, and grass-fed butter.
- Include supplements that will help with antioxidants and healing.
- Eat foods that detox and repair your body like cruciferous vegetables and garlic.
- Have protein with every meal to help keep your blood sugar balanced.

Changing your diet may feel like you are restricting your choices in the beginning, especially if the foods you enjoy right now aren't on this liver-approved list. What's important to remember is that you are doing this for you, for your future self, for your health, and for all the people who want you in their life. Right now there are things you'd like to do, places to go, and goals that need to be accomplished. Healing your liver and reversing NAFLD will help you get there, allowing you to pursue what you want with a healthy body, more energy, and a better-functioning liver. Don't look at changing your diet as something that you're being forced into, rather choose to look at this as an opportunity to become a healthier, stronger version of yourself—one that is equipped with the strength to make their goals happen! That being said, it's important to eliminate saturated fats, excess sodium, refined sugars, and fructose from your diet as much as possible, as all of these substances are harmful to your liver and will perpetuate the negative cycle and side effects of NAFLD.

Change Your Lifestyle

There are a number of lifestyle changes not related to diet that are important to make for the health of your liver. Giving up smoking and drinking, working to improve your mindset, and taking up an exercise routine are all important aspects of managing or reversing NAFLD. As we already talked about, including daily exercise for at least 30 minutes every day will improve your metabolism and decrease insulin resistance. However, the key to adjusting your lifestyle doesn't just lie in having a different diet or a specific exercise plan. It comes from moving more on a regular basis, taking part in activities that get you up and moving either inside your home or outside on an adventure. Simple things like walking to your closest coffee shop, parking farther away when you go to the store, taking the stairs instead of the elevator, and switching out cocktails with water on a regular occasion, will all help aid the reversal of fatty liver disease.

You may find that eliminating obvious things like drugs and alcohol in the beginning while you are still working to reverse NAFLD or NASH will make the process happen faster. It could be that being strict with your diet plan is something that can be more flexible in the future, so look at forgoing these items with that in mind. There's no guarantee that your liver will once again be happy eating these foods and be effective in digesting them, but don't focus on that for now. Look instead to the here and now, the changes you need to make to have an overall healthier, more active lifestyle that restricts or limits the kinds of foods your body has a hard time processing or absorbing. In time, cravings for those things may disappear entirely as you find new, healthy behaviors and habits to replace bad habits or poor diet choices.

Consider Alternative Medicines

While alternative medical practices cannot replace traditional medicine, and while it's essential to listen to the advice of your primary physician throughout your entire treatment, alternative or complementary medicine can be a helpful part of your individualized treatment plan. This can include whole medicine practices such as traditional Chinese medicine, or energy-based approaches like reiki. The options are endless, so do some research to help you decide whether you could benefit from incorporating alternative medicine into your liver health regimen. Don't be afraid to advocate for yourself if you'd like to include alternative or complementary medicinal treatments because it may be something that works well for you. With your doctor's approval in mind, there's no limit to the kinds of alternative medicines you can incorporate into your overall plan to reverse fatty liver disease.

It's good to note that managing your stress is something that is beneficial in more ways than only healing your liver. By regularly releasing stress, moving that tension out of your body, and addressing things in your life that feel overwhelming, cause anxiety, or trigger depression, you'll be a much healthier person. It will also help you avoid binging on or craving sugary or processed foods. Our emotions play a huge role in what foods our mind tells us to seek out, as each type of food has an energetic quality and emotional impact on our body and mind. Alternative medicine that emphasizes detoxing your body from negativity, removes emotional or physical toxicity, and promotes overall well-being, balance, and mental health can only help you on your journey of healing your liver and reversing NAFLD or NASH.

Consider Herbal Supplements

While there are no currently approved pharmacological interventions for NAFLD, scientific research shows that supplementing with extracts of certain herbs and other plants can benefit the health of your liver. It is crucial that you check with your doctor before taking any herbal supplements since some of them have been connected to liver damage. That being said, some may have benefits that could help your liver and can be added into your meal plan with your doctor's approval.

Here is a list herbs that have shown healing properties for the liver:

- Milk thistle can have a strong antioxidant impact on the body.
- Ginseng has anti-inflammatory properties and can protect against liver injury.
- Green tea may protect the body against further liver damage.
- Licorice, not the candy version, is used in Chinese and Japanese medicine.
- Turmeric can reduce inflammation in the body.
- Garlic has liver-protecting properties and can boost liver health.

- Ginger may reduce inflammation and liver damage, and lower cholesterol.
- Danshen can protect against disease and stimulate liver tissue regeneration.
- Ginkgo biloba may increase liver function.
- Astragalus has been shown to protect the liver when used with other herbs.

Although some of these may work together to help support the healing of your liver, be cautious when ingesting them and talk to your doctor before self-prescribing them to your diet. Everybody has a different body and genetic makeup, which means some herbs may have adverse side effects or create more damage to your liver. They may also become toxic to you if you have preexisting conditions, and can sometimes be contaminated with heavy metals, pharmaceuticals, pesticides, and bacteria that might cause more harm than good. If you are going to add herbal supplements into your diet, do your research into how the herb is farmed, packaged, and what it contains. Read the labels and learn about the business you are buying from to find the best, organic, and cleanest option of that herb you want. These supplements can work to fight oxidative stress, reduce inflammation, and boost your liver's natural defenses against fat buildup. However, since not all herbal supplements are appropriate for everyone, proceed with caution and consume everything in moderation, staying in touch with your doctor as you include herbal supplements in your treatment plan.

Conclusion

Since we've now addressed virtually every aspect of managing NAFLD, we'll keep the conclusion short to avoid boring you with repetition! After finishing this book, you are now much more equipped with the knowledge you need to have about your condition than before you started. You've learned all about the different parts of the liver, how it functions, and some of the things that can damage it, in terms that will allow you to communicate your concerns to your doctor and other medical professionals. Learning about the liver empowers you to take control of your treatment, by helping you fully understand what's happening to your body and what needs to be done to fix it. The liver is an important part of your body and needs to be taken care of, just like everything else. Sometimes we take for granted that the liver regularly detoxifies our bodies, helps digest difficult foods, and works in our favor to keep our body functioning at its highest level. When you understand why the liver is here and the vital role it plays in your life, you may anewfound respect forming for the organ. We've also prepared you to go through the diagnostic process by outlining the common tests that are performed when a doctor suspects liver problems, and what to expect from them. Running tests is not a scary process, or at least it shouldn't be, but rather is your chance to get a clearer understanding of what's happening underneath the surface and how you need to address any problems that are found. We've gone over the lifestyle changes that your physician may recommend as part of your treatment, as well as how you can put these into practice. Your diet, actions that promote weight loss, and a general increase of activity will all play a key role in reversing fatty liver disease. Fortunately, the recommended diet follows a Mediterranean meal plan, which is one that is filled with thousands of delicious dishes of a wide variety so you'll never feel bored or like you've been missing out on eating interesting things. Stay curious and open to new spices, flavor combinations, and types of meals you can eat to keep food fun, interesting, and appetizing.

Changing your habits can be simple when you approach it with the mindset of healing your body, and giving it the rest and changes it deserves to be healthy again. Small steps in the right direction will all add up to big change that will positively impact your present self and future you. Finally, we've explored herbal supplements and other alternative medical practices that you may find beneficial when it comes to managing your fatty liver disease. It was our hope when writing this book that you will be able to use this knowledge to take the reins of your treatment, and to work towards a better, healthier lifestyle for yourself and your liver. The most important thing to remember, which we've reiterated throughout the book, is that your liver will be as good to you as you are to it. Your best chance at reversing or successfully managing NAFLD is to catch it early and make the required lifestyle changes to turn it around. Don't forget that you are in control, and your motivation in following through with your treatment plan is of the utmost importance.

You might be reading this book because you suspect you have NAFLD or another liver condition, because you've already been diagnosed, or you are simply interested in the topic of liver health. If you think you have NAFLD, it's important to get your symptoms checked out as soon as possible to stop the disease from progressing any further. If you've been diagnosed, now is the time to start making the lifestyle changes required to get your liver health back on track. If you don't have any experience with NAFLD, this book can still be helpful in identifying risk factors and making preemptive lifestyle changes that help prevent the disease from developing in the first place.

Your liver is your best friend when it comes to maintaining the health of your body. In appreciation for all it does, as well as to keep it functioning in top shape, it's essential to treat your liver well. It deserves it! Now that you've read this book, you're armed with the knowledge you need to start taking better care of your liver today. Use everything you have learned to make any necessary changes to your lifestyle and diet, starting with what your doctor recommends and then building out from there. Making adjustments will be very beneficial, not only for your liver, but for your overall health and can help you enjoy a better future and life.

References

American Heart Association. (n.d.). Saturated fat. https://www.heart.org/en/healthy-living/healthy-eating/eat-smart/fats/saturated-fats

American Liver Foundation. (2021, March 26). Liver disease diets. https://liverfoundation.org/for-patients/about-the-liver/health-wellness/nutrition/

American Liver Foundation. (2022, January 21). NASH symptoms. https://liverfoundation.org/for-patients/about-the-liver/diseases-of-the-liver/nonalcoholic-steatohepatitis-information-center/nash-symptoms/

American Liver Foundation. (2022, January 12). The progression of liver disease. https://liverfoundation.org/for-patients/about-the-liver/the-progression-of-liver-disease

Barhum, L. (2018, August 7). What are the health benefits of goji berries? Medical News Today. https://www.medicalnewstoday.com/articles/322693

https://www.medicalnewstoday.com/articles/322693 Bouazza, A., Bitam, A., Amiali, M., Bounihi, A., Yargui, L., & Koceir, E. A. (2015). Effect of fruit vinegars on liver damage and oxidative stress in high-fat-fed rats. Pharmaceutical Biology, 54(2), 260–265. https://doi.org/10.3109/13880209.2015.1031910

Burke, D., & Rossiaky, D. (2021, December 14). Aspartate aminotransferase (AST) test. Healthline. https://www.healthline.com/health/ast#uses

Cai, L., Wan, D., Yi, F., & Luan, L. (2017). Purification, preliminary characterization and hepatoprotective effects of polysaccharides from dandelion root. Molecules, 22(9), 1409. https://doi.org/10.3390/molecules22091409

Canadian Liver Foundation. (n.d.-a). Liver diseases. https://www.liver.ca/patients-caregivers/liver-diseases/

Centers for Disease Control and Prevention. (n.d.-b). Adult obesity facts. https://www.cdc.gov/obesity/data/adult.html

Centers for Disease Control and Prevention (n.d.-c). Hepatitis A information. https://www.cdc.gov/hepatitis/hav/index.htm

Centers for Disease Control and Prevention. (n.d.-d). Hepatitis B information. https://www.cdc.gov/hepatitis/hbv/index.htm

Centers for Disease Control and Prevention. (n.d.-e). Hepatitis C information. https://www.cdc.gov/hepatitis/hcv/index.htm

Centers for Disease Control and Prevention. (n.d.-f). Hepatitis D information. https://www.cdc.gov/hepatitis/hdv/index.htm

Choi, Y., Lee, J. E., Chang, Y., Kim, M. K., Sung, E., Shin, H., & Ryu, S. (2016). Dietary sodium and potassium intake in relation to non-alcoholic fatty liver disease. The British Journal of Nutrition, 116(8), 1447–1456. https://doi.org/10.1017/S0007114516003391

Choresand, T. (n.d.). Best diet for non alcoholic fatty liver disease—Cure your fatty liver naturally (for good!). Terpsi Choresand. https://terpsichoresand.org/best-diet-for-non-alcoholic-fatty-liver-disease-cure-your-fatty-liver-naturally-for-good/

Cicero, A. F. G., Colletti, A., & Bellentani, S. (2018). Nutraceutical approach to non-alcoholic fatty liver disease (NAFLD): The available clinical evidence. Nutrients, 10(9), 1153. https://doi.org/10.3390/nu10091153

CleanseJoy. (2019, January 1). Liver detox drink: Evidence based recipe for liver & gallbladder. CleanseJoy: Evidence Based Cleansing. https://cleansejoy.com/liver-detox-drink/

Clear, J. (2018). Atomic habits: An easy & proven way to build good habits & break bad ones. Avery.

Clifford, T., Howatson, G., West, D. J., & Stevenson, E. J. (2015). The potential benefits of red beetroot supplementation in health and disease. Nutrients, 7(4), 2801–2822. https://doi.org/10.3390/nu7042801

Clouthier, S. (n.d.). These 8 pillars of holistic health will keep you in balance. Alternative Health Center of the Woodlands. https://ahcwoodlands.com/these-8-pillars-of-holistic-health-will-keep-you-in-balance/

Creswell, J. D., Taren, A A., Lindsay, E. K., Greco, C. M., Gianaros, P. J., Fairgrieve, A., Marsland, A. L., Brown, K. W., Way, B. M., Rosen, R. K., & Ferris, J. L. (2016). Alterations in resting-state functional connectivity link mindfulness meditation with reduced interleukin-6: A randomized controlled trial. Biological Psychiatry, 80(1), 53–61. https://doi.org/10.1016/j.biopsych.2016.01.008

Ecowatch. (2016, May 7). 7 ways to heal a fatty liver. https://www.ecowatch.com/7-ways-to-heal-a-fatty-liver-1891128750.html

Farhana, A., & Lappin, S. L. (2021, May 7). Biochemistry, lactate dehydrogenase. StatPearls Publishing. https://www.ncbi.nlm.nih.gov/books/NBK557536/

Fatty Liver Disease. (2021, August 4). Maintaining liver health: How to lower liver enzymes. https://fattyliverdisease.com/how-to-lower-liver-enzymes/

Fletcher, J. (2021, February 25). What is hydrogenated oil and is it safe? Medical News Today. https://www.medicalnewstoday.com/articles/hydrogentated-oil

Foo, J. (2018, May). Liver condition improved after 9 months of Tai Chi. Hua Ying Wushu & Tai Chi Academy. https://davidbao.com/2018/05/30/evident-health-benefit/

Gao, S. (2017, March 10). Traditional Chinese medicine tricks to detox your liver. Culture Trip. https://theculturetrip.com/asia/china/articles/traditional-chinese-medicine-tricks-to-detox-your-liver/

Garbar, V., & Newton, B. W. (2021, July 26). Anatomy, abdomen and pelvis, falciform ligament. StatPearls Publishing. https://www.ncbi.nlm.nih.gov/books/NBK539858/

Garlick, P. (2004). The nature of human hazards associated with excessive intake of amino acids. *The Journal of Nutrition*, 134(6), 1633S-1639S. https://doi.org/10.1093/jn/134.6.1633S

Genetic and Rare Diseases Information Center. (2012, February 24). *Nonalcoholic steatohepatitis.* https://rarediseases.info.nih.gov/diseases/6430/nonalcoholic-steatohepatitis

Gurarie, M. (2022, February 24). *Anatomy of the hepatic veins.* Verywell Health. https://www.verywellhealth.com/hepatic-veins-anatomy-4782649

Gyimah, A. (2021, July 16). *Can you eat fruit with nonalcoholic fatty liver disease (NAFLD)?* Clean Eating. https://www.cleaneatingmag.com/clean-diet/disease-prevention/can-you-eat-fruit-with-nonalcoholic-fatty-liver-disease-nafld/

Harvard Health Publishing. (2019). *Positive psychology: Harnessing the power of happiness, mindfulness, and inner strength.* Harvard Medical School. https://www.health.harvard.edu/mind-and-mood/positive-psychology-harnessing-the-power-of-happiness-mindfulness-and-inner-strength#about-report

Healthline Editorial Team. (2018a, January 20). Hepatic artery proper. Healthline. https://www.healthline.com/human-body-maps/hepatic-artery-proper#1

Healthline Editorial Team. (2018b, January 20). Hepatic veins. Healthline. https://www.healthline.com/human-body-maps/hepatic-veins

Healthline Editorial Team. (2018c, January 22). Common hepatic duct. Healthline. https://www.healthline.com/human-body-maps/common-hepatic-duct#1

Johns Hopkins Medicine. (n.d.). Diet for fatty liver disease. https://www.hopkinsmedicine.org/endoscopic-weight-loss-program/conditions/fatty_liver_disease.html

Johnson J. (2018, January 12). Are fructooligosaccharides safe? Medical News Today. https://www.medicalnewstoday.com/articles/319299

Jones, T. (2019, September 29). 11 foods that are good for your liver. Healthline. https://www.healthline.com/nutrition/11-foods-for-your-liver

Kakleas, K., Christodouli, F., & Karavanaki, K. (2020, March 6). Nonalcoholic fatty liver disease, insulin resistance, and sweeteners: A literature review. Expert Review of Endocrinology & Metabolism, 15(2) 83-93. https://doi.org/10.1080/17446651.2020.1740588

Krajka-Kuźniak, V., Szaefer, H., Ignatowicz, E., Adamska, T., Markowski, J., & Baer-Dubowska, W. (2015). Influence of cloudy apple juice on N-nitrosodiethylamine-induced liver injury and phases I and II biotransformation enzymes in rat liver. Acta Poloniae Pharmaceutica, 72(2), 267–276. https://pubmed.ncbi.nlm.nih.gov/26642677/

Kriel, G. (2021, February 4). Holistic medicine: A beginner's guide. Thumos Health Center. https://www.thumoshealthcenter.com/holistic-medicine-a-beginners-guide/

Krishnamurthy, M. S. (n.d.). Lemon uses, juice benefits, home remedies. Easy Ayurveda. https://www.easyayurveda.com/2012/11/14/health-benefits-of-lemon-ayurveda-details/#medicinal_properties

Lambert, J. E., Parnell, J. A., Eksteen, B., Raman, M., Bomhof, M. R., Rioux, K. P., Madsen, K. L., & Reimer, R. A. (2015). Gut microbiota manipulation with prebiotics in patients with non-alcoholic fatty liver disease: A randomized controlled trial protocol. BMC Gastroenterology, 15(169). https://doi.org/10.1186/s12876-015-0400-5

Liu, T., Yang, L.-L., Zou, L., Li, D.-F., Wen, H.-Z., Zheng, P.-Y., Xing, L.-J., Song, H.-Y., Tang, X.-D., & Ji, G. (2013). Evidence-based complementary and alternative medicine, 2013. https://doi.org/10.1155/2013/429738

Liu, X., Miller, Y. D., Burton, N. W., & Brown, W. J. (2008). A preliminary study of the effects of Tai Chi and Qigong medical exercise on indicators of metabolic syndrome, glycaemic control, health-related quality of life, and psychological health in adults with elevated blood glucose. *British Journal of Sports Medicine, 44*(10), 704–709. https://doi.org/10.1136/bjsm.2008.051144

Liz. (2018, November 22). Qigong for the liver. Qigong Exercises for Beginners. https://qigongexercisesforbeginners.com/qigong-for-the-liver

Loverling, C. (2021, November 5). Alkaline phosphatase level (ALP) test. Healthline. https://www.healthline.com/health/alp

Mahesh, M., Bharathi, M., Reddy, M. R. G., Kumar, M. S., Putcha, U. K., Vajreswari, A., & Jeyakumar, S. M. (2016). Carrot juice administration decreases liver stearoyl-CoA desaturase 1 and improves docosahexaenoic acid levels, but not steatosis in high fructose diet-fed weanling Wistar rats. *Preventive Nutrition and Food Science, 21*(3), 171–180. https://doi.org/10.3746/pnf.2016.21.3.171

Marchione, V. (2016, October 10). Bile function and liver: Foods that help increase bile production. Bel Marra Health. https://www.belmarrahealth.com/bile-function-liver-foods-help-increase-bile-production/

Martin, D. (2019, September 29). How to perform a liver cleanse with Ayurveda. Svastha Ayurveda. https://svasthaayurveda.com/how-to-perform-a-liver-cleanse-with-ayurveda/

Mayo Clinic. (n.d.). Bilirubin test. https://www.mayoclinic.org/tests-procedures/bilirubin/about/pac-20393041

Mayo Clinic. (n.d.). Biofeedback. https://www.mayoclinic.org/tests-procedures/biofeedback/about/pac-20384664

Mayo Clinic. (n.d.). CT scan. Mayo Clinic. https://www.mayoclinic.org/tests-procedures/ct-scan/about/pac-20393675

Medline Plus. (2020a, July 30). Albumi*n blood test.* National Library of Medicine. https://medlineplus.gov/lab-tests/albumin-blood-test/

Medline Plus. (2020b, July 30). *ALT blood test.* National Library of Medicine. https://medlineplus.gov/lab-tests/alt-blood-test/

Medline Plus. (2020c, December 17). *Lactate dehydrogenase (LDH) test.* National Library of Medicine. https://medlineplus.gov/lab-tests/lactate-dehydrogenase-ldh-test/

Medline Plus. (2021a, September 9). *Elastography.* National Library of Medicine. https://medlineplus.gov/lab-tests/elastography/

Medline Plus. (2021b, November 16). *Gamma-glutamyl transferase (GGT) test.* National Library of Medicine. https://medlineplus.gov/lab-tests/gamma-glutamyl-transferase-ggt-test/

Merkes, M. (2010). Mindfulness-based stress reduction for people with chronic diseases. *Australian Journal of Primary Health, 16*(3), 200-210. https://doi.org/10.1071/py09063

Mir, H. M., Stepanova, M., Afendy, H., Cable, R., & Younossi, Z. M. (2013). Association of sleep disorders with nonalcoholic fatty liver disease (NAFLD): A population-based study. *Journal of Clinical and Experimental Hepatology, 3*(3), 181-185. https://doi.org/10.1016/j.jceh.2013.06.004

Modaresi Esfeh, J., & Ansari-Gilani, K. (2015). Steatosis and hepatitis C. *Gastroenterology Report, 4*(1) 24-29. https://doi.org/10.1093/gastro/gov040

Moll, J. (2021, December 26). *The difference between saturated and unsaturated fats.* Verywell Health. https://www.verywellhealth.com/difference-between-saturated-fats-and-unsaturated-fats-697517

Morstein, M. (2010, January 6). *Non-alcoholic fatty liver disease*. Naturopathic Doctor News and Review. https://ndnr.com/pain-medicine/jan-non-alcoholic-fatty-liver-disease/

Nagy, L. (2012). Would eating carrots protect your liver? A new role involving NKT cells for retinoic acid in hepatitis. *European Journal of Immunology, 42*(7), 1677–1680. https://doi.org/10.1002/eji.201242705

Nall, R. (2022, January 24). *The liver*. Healthline. https://www.healthline.com/human-body-maps/liver

The NASH Education Program. (n.d.). *How prevalent is NASH?* https://www.the-nash-education-program.com/what-is-nash/how-prevalent-is-nash/

National Center for Complementary and Integrative Health. (2020, April). *Dandelion*. https://www.nccih.nih.gov/health/dandelion

National Institute of Diabetes and Digestive and Kidney Issues. (n.d.). *Eating, diet, & nutrition for NAFLD & NASH*. https://www.niddk.nih.gov/health-information/liver-disease/nafld-nash/eating-diet-nutrition

Nazıroğlu, M., Güler, M., Özgül, C., Saydam, G., Küçükayaz, M., & Sözbir, E. (2014). Apple cider vinegar modulates serum lipid profile, erythrocyte, kidney, and liver membrane oxidative stress in ovariectomized mice fed high cholesterol. *The Journal of Membrane Biology, 247*(8), 667–673. https://doi.org/10.1007/s00232-014-9685-5

NHLBI Obesity Education Initiative Expert Panel on the Identification, Evaluation, and Treatment of Obesity in Adults (US). (1998). *Clinical guidelines on the identification, evaluation, and treatment of overweight and obesity in adults: The evidence report*. National Heart, Lung, and Blood Institute. https://www.ncbi.nlm.nih.gov/books/NBK2009/

Perdomo, C. M., Fruhbeck, G., & Escalada, J. (2019). Impact of nutritional changes on nonalcoholic fatty liver disease. *Nutrients, 11*(3), 677. https://doi.org/10.3390/nu11030677

Perumpail, B. J., Li, A. A., Iqbal, U., Sallam, S., Shah, N. D., Kwong, W., Cholankeril, G., Kim, D., & Ahmed, A. (2018). Potential therapeutic benefits of herbs and supplements in patients with NAFLD. *Diseases, 6*(3), 80. https://doi.org/10.3390/diseases6030080

Pfizer Medical Team. (2018, September 20). *What you need to know about this silent liver disease called NASH*. Get Healthy, Stay Healthy. https://www.gethealthystayhealthy.com/articles/what-you-need-to-know-about-this-silent-liver-disease-called-nash

The pitta type in Ayurveda. (n.d.). Somatheeram Ayurvedic Health Resort. https://somatheeram.org/en/pitta/

RadiologyInfo.org (n.d.). *Magnetic resonance cholangiopancreatography (MRCP)*. https://www.radiologyinfo.org/en/info/mrcp

Rahimlou, M., Yari, Z., Hekmatdoost, A., Alavian, S. M., & Keshavarz, S. A. (2016). Ginger supplementation in nonalcoholic fatty liver disease: A randomized, double-blind, placebo-controlled pilot study. *Hepatitis Monthly, 16*(1). https://doi.org/10.5812/hepatmon.34897

Ramesh, S., & Sanyal, A. J. (2004). Hepatitis C and nonalcoholic fatty liver disease. *Seminars in Liver Disease, 24*(4), 399–413. https://doi.org/10.1055/s-2004-860869

Raypole, C. (2021, November 18). *Liver problems and their causes*. Healthline. https://www.healthline.com/health/liver-diseases

Printed in Great Britain
by Amazon